BAD BACKS
and
PAINFUL PARTS

Jenny Draspa M.C.S.P.

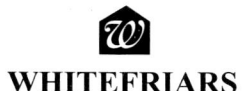

WHITEFRIARS

BAD BACKS

and
PAINFUL NECKS
PAINFUL ELBOWS
PAINFUL SHOULDERS
PAINFUL CHEST WALLS
PAINFUL RIBS
PAINFUL GROINS
PAINFUL LEGS

This book is written by
Jenny Draspa,
Chartered Physiotherapist.

It is based on her clinical experience which has been built up in her private practice and developed from the research by her late husband, Leon J. Draspa.

His research was awarded a Ph.D. from Edinburgh University.

Copyright Jennifer Draspa 1996

Published by Whitefriars, Whitefriars House, Whitefriars, Chester. CH1 1NZ.

All rights reserved. No part of this work may be reproduced nor may it be stored in an information retrieval system (other than short extracts for purposes of review) without the express permission of the Publishers given in writing.

ISBN 0 9527326 0 2

ACKNOWLEDGEMENTS

My special thanks must go to Michael Ashton for his valuable assistance in editing and clarifying my manuscript for this book.

The picture on page 13 has previously been printed in 'Manwatching', by Desmond Morris, published by Triad Panther, (1978). The picture of the faces was taken by Dr. Morris from a book entitled 'The Art of Pantomime', by Charles Aubert, (1927), no publisher given.

The cartoon of the two men, 'Familiarity breeds contempt', on page 14, is by H.M. Bateman. Copyright © H.M. Bateman 1969. It is taken from Michael Bateman's 'The man who drew the 20th Century', published by Macdonald in 1969.

The other fifty four pictures and anatomical drawings were drawn by Anthony Lewis, Steve Martin and Shawn Stipling.

Artists

Shawn Stipling. Figures, C, D, E, F(i-iii), G(i-iii), H, I, K(ii), L, M(i-ii), N(i), O, P, Q, R(i-v), S(i-vi), X(v).

Steve Martin. Figures, J(i-ii), K(i), T(i-iii), U(i-iii), V(i-ii), W(i), X(i-iv).

Anthony Lewis. Figures, T(iv), U(iv-v), V(iii), W(ii), X(vi).

Foreword

Backache, and other common and widespread aches and pains in the body, which can cause such discomfort and concern to sufferers, have long been thought to be caused by pressure on a nerve.

However, it is now realised by anatomists (Bogduk, N. and Twomey, L.T. *See Bibliography*) and physiologists, that pressure on a nerve produces paralysis or anaesthesia. It does not produce the aching pain that is the symptom of backache and the other continuing and inexplicable aches and pains that we experience.

This aching pain is produced in the muscles by muscle tension over a considerable period of time which stimulates the specialised nerves within the muscles. For practitioners, these nerves are called the Golgi tendon organs.

The muscle tension is not always visible and it is outside our conscious control.

The cause of the muscle tension is Body Language. Body Language is a reflex and can be a continual postural reaction caused by our emotions, which themselves are a reaction to circumstances we find ourselves in.

Our emotions are provoked by stress.

This book defines stress and shows its link to Body Language.

It describes Body Language and shows its effect. Diagrams and pictures of muscles and posture, show clearly which muscles are affected.

Finally, it advises the patient on how, having identified the Body Language and muscle problems, they should approach the pain and finally get rid of it.

The book is written for the layman. However, the anatomy, the link between stress and Body Language, and the mechanism of Body Language producing pain, will be of interest to Chartered Physiotherapists, other therapists working in this field, and G.P's.

Contents

8   **How to use this book**

PART 1 NECKS AND BACKS

9   *Chapter 1*
INTRODUCTION TO BAD BACKS AND PAINFUL PARTS
Muscles – Muscle tension – Pain – Stress

10 *Chapter 2*
PAIN AND MUSCLES
Use of muscles by sportsmen, and normal everyday use – Tense muscles – 'Slipped discs'.

12 *Chapter 3*
STRESS
What is meant by stress – Who it affects.

13 *Chapter 4*
BODY LANGUAGE
What is meant by Body Language – Facial expressions – Body movements.

15 *Chapter 5*
STRESS ⟶ PAIN
How can stress produce pain – Why is the pain sometimes in the back? – Why is the pain sometimes in the neck?

18 *Chapter 6*
MUSCLES
Muscles tense when emotions are affected – Only part of a muscle can be tense and still look normal – The whole muscle can tense and affect posture – Very tense neck muscles. Very tense back muscles.

19 *Chapter 7*
REFERRED PAIN
What is referred pain – Muscles involved.

20 *Chapter 8*
CHANGES IN PAIN
Why does pain move sometimes? – Fluctuations of pain – Anxiety.

21 *Chapter 9*
PAIN AND THE NERVE RECEPTORS Anatomy of pain in muscles – Trigger spots – Golgi tendon organs.

22 *Chapter 10*
TREATMENT TO NECKS AND BACKS
Treatment of painful muscle by patient – Heat – Massage – Relaxation – Breathing – Treatment of painful muscle by chartered physiotherapist.

26 *Chapter 11*
TREATMENT OF STRESS
How to get rid of the cause – the stress itself.

27 *Chapter 12*
SUMMARY
Stress – Emotions – Body Language – Muscles – Muscle tension – Pain.

28 *Chapter 13*
PHYSICAL SUPPORT FOR THE NECK AND THE BACK
In bed with neck pain – In bed with backache – Sitting on a chair with backache – Lumbar rolls – D.I.Y. Lumbar rolls.

31 *Chapter 14*
    EXAMPLES OF STRESS AND THE MAIN MUSCLES INVOLVED
    Stress affecting the neck – Stress affecting the back.

33 *Chapter 15*
    MUSCLES INVOLVED
    In the neck and head and in the back and the back of the leg – Pictures of the muscles – The muscles' main actions – Painful everyday actions and hints on how to minimise the pain – Simple exercises – Muscles in referred pain.

40 *Chapter 16*
    EMERGENCIES
    I'm at the boot of the car – I'm stuck! What do I do? – Picking up a parcel from the floor – I'm stuck! What do I do?

PART 2
OTHER PAINFUL PARTS

43 *Chapter 17*
    INTRODUCTION TO PART 2

44 *Chapter 18*
    TENNIS ELBOW and GOLFER'S ELBOW
    What is it? – Muscles involved – Pictures – Treatment – The cause – Examples

49 *Chapter 19*
    PAIN IN THE SHOULDER
    What is it? – Muscles involved – Pictures – Treatment – The cause – Examples

53 *Chapter 20*
    PAIN IN THE CHEST WALL
    What is it? – Muscles involved – Pictures – Treatment– The cause – Examples

56 *Chapter 21*
    PAIN IN THE FRONT OF THE RIBS
    What is it? – Muscle involved – Pictures – Treatment – The cause – Examples

59 *Chapter 22*
    PAIN IN THE GROIN AND THE FRONT OF THE THIGHS
    What is it? – Muscles involved – Pictures – Treatment – The cause – Examples

60 *Chapter 23*
    MASSAGE
    Why do we massage the muscles? – How do we do it? – Preparation of the patient – Preparation of the masseur – What are the actual massage movements?

68 *Chapter 24*
    QUESTIONS

70 *Chapter 25*
    SUMMARY

71 **How to use this book**

72 **Bibliography**

How to use this book

The book covers most parts of the body.

To get the full understanding of the sequence by which pain is the result of muscle tension, caused by Body Language, which itself is the result of stress, first read chapters 1 to 12. This will greatly help you in dealing with your specific problem. It is true that chapters 1 to 12 talk about pain in the neck and back only. Don't let this put you off. The mechanism as to how the pain is produced applies to backs and necks and to other parts of the body. So read these chapters first, and then the chapter that particularly interests you.

For example: if tennis elbow is the problem, read chapters 1 to 12, then read the chapter on tennis elbow. So for:

Necks and Backs	Chapters 1 to 16
Tennis Elbow	Chapters 1 to 12 then Chapters 17 and 18
Shoulder	Chapters 1 to 12 then Chapters 17 and 19
Chest wall	Chapters 1 to 12 then Chapters 17 and 20
Front of the ribs	Chapters 1 to 12 then Chapters 17 and 21
Front of the thighs and groin	Chapters 1 to 12 then Chapters 17 and 22

Then finally, read the Sumary in Chapter 25.

PART I
NECKS and BACKS

Chapter 1
Introduction

People fill the doctors' surgeries with what they describe as a 'neck' or a 'back pain', or more specifically doctors describe it as spondylosis, narrowed disc spaces, 'slipped disc', lumbar strain, fibrositis etc., etc. Confusingly, one patient may be given three different diagnoses from three different doctors for a similar condition. A patient may even be told by the doctor that "nothing is wrong", but what he means is that there is no disease or structural damage. However the patients do not always understand how this can be, especially as they are in pain. Whatever the diagnosis, they rarely get sympathy from their friends and relatives!

This book will describe how the pain people suffer, in the neck and back and in other areas, can be due to muscle tension, that is tension in a precise muscle or muscle group. Muscles become tense due to stress. When these muscles *remain tense*, they become painful. The book will show that the pain, which 'just comes on', as people say, commences at the start of a stress situation and will vary in intensity as the stress varies. It will describe in detail the physical treatment necessary for the painful muscles. It will show that the pain clears up and will not re-occur, *only* when

a) the stress stops; or

b) the patient changes his attitude so that it is no longer a stress to him; or

c) the patient forgets the stress.

Of course, *any person in pain should always consult a doctor and have the cause diagnosed*. If the doctor diagnoses it as a pain in the muscles due to stress, treatment of the muscles is necessary, and counselling for the stress condition may be helpful in some cases.

Chapter 2
Pain and Muscles

When we have pain, described as neck ache or back ache, we can certainly feel it but sometimes we're not very good at localising it. We cannot always put our fingers right on the spot, right on the source of pain. However, this book will show you how it can be localised to a muscle, or to several muscles.

A funny thing about muscles is that although they play such an important part in our lives we are not all that interested in them. Well, a few people are – the body builders and the sportsmen. The rest of us are aware of them only when they are stiff and painful after we have over-used them; like the day after we have played the season's first hard game of squash; or the day after we have dug the garden over at our new house.

Body builders and sportsmen generally, are aware of their muscles. Footballers and runners will all know their Hamstring muscles (which are at the back of the thigh), because they or their friends, may well have injured them. Non sporty people probably know the bulging muscle on Popeye's arm.

Muscles are what we call the flesh of our bodies. Body builders develop them to show them off. Maybe we don't want to show them off, but we all need to move. It is muscles that make us move when we run after a bus or play the piano, or perform any movement at all.

When we move, a muscle is made to work. To do so, it becomes shorter and harder. It is contracting and tensing. When a muscle becomes shorter, it moves the bones and so the limbs and the body move. All this movement of the muscles is consciously controlled by us. We know we want to move an arm, run for a bus or play the piano. In normal circumstances these actions are not painful.

However, muscles can also contract, or tense, *without* our control, when we are *not* moving. Muscles which are tense are not, at first, painful. However, it is when they *remain tense* that they become painful. It is when this happens that these muscles cause pain in the neck and backache; pain which may be exceedingly severe.

Quite often these tense muscles may be visible. When the whole muscle is tense it 'stands out'. On the other hand, it may only be part of a muscle which is tense, so it does not 'stand out', and it looks normal.

The pain is predominantly of an aching variety, whether it be short sharp stabs or a prolonged dull ache.

When people suffer from pain in their backs, they think of 'slipped discs'. "It is so painful, it must be a disc," they say. They cannot believe that muscles could be so painful. But they can. Think of cramp. When you have cramp, you cannot think of anything else! We are not discussing cramp here, but it does show just how painful muscles can become.

By 'slipped disc', it is meant that the disc has slipped and is putting pressure on a nerve. However, pressure on a nerve does not produce aching pain; it produces, temporarily, or ultimately permanent, paralysis or loss of normal sensation. Think what happens when you sit on your hands or legs. Your hand or leg becomes numb. Think what happens when you are sitting and you cross your legs. The knees press on a nerve and your foot 'goes dead'. It may be uncomfortable but it does not hurt.

We are talking about aching pain – the aching pain of neck and backache.

These tense and painful muscles causing neck and back pain can be made even more tense, such as when we turn our head, or when we bend down to pick something up, and therefore become even more painful. When however, with treatment, we can relax the muscles, the pain goes.

"Well that's fine," you may say, "but why did it come on in the first place?"

"It came on because of stress".

"Stress?" you query.

"Stress".

"But," you may ask, "I haven't got any excessive pressures. I am quite a capable person. I don't have stress, and on occasions when I do, I cope with it quite easily."

"Generally this is true, but there are times when we can't cope."

"Well anyway, how could stress, which is abstract, produce pain?"

"It can and it does, and this book will explain how. Before it does that, however, we need to define stress."

Chapter 3
Stress

Stress is a much over used word which, unfortunately, means different things to different people. To some, it means losing one's job, losing one's loved ones, a child involved in an accident, the house burning down.

To others it can mean answering six telephones under pressure, having a job where you are at everyone's beck and call, having too many commitments, being committed to others for most hours of every day and most days of every week.

What is important to remember is that *stress is individually determined*. Working seven days a week, answering six telephones and being at everybodys' beck and call may be stress to one person (even a nightmare!) but to another, maybe the elixir of life. Losing a relative may be a stress ('the end of the world') to one person; to another, even if not dancing with joy, it may leave them unmoved.

Perhaps the most important thing about defining stress is that there is no one kind of stress. It is *always* individually determined. It is stress to you as an individual. After all, you are an individual, you are not a group to be categorised.

Stress, in this case, means anything which interferes with the happiness and contentment of a person or with the smooth running of their life; anything which interferes with their wishes or aspirations; anything which 'needles' them; anything which upsets the equilibrium of their life.

It can affect anybody in any walk of life.

Stress to one person is frequently not seen or understood by other people because that person does not necessarily tell other people what they are thinking, or what they are feeling. We don't tell everybody our innermost thoughts.

How is it that people, nice people, who are calm, capable, non hysterical, well able to hold down difficult jobs, well able to cope with different kinds of crises, well able to carry responsibilities, and who are described and admired by their friends and colleagues as calm and capable, can suffer? How could *those* people suffer from stress? On the face of it, it seems rather unlikely.

There is a feeling amongst the general public that it is the emotional, histrionic people who may suffer stress, but certainly not the ones who are able to keep control of themselves and who, in all adversity, manage to keep 'a stiff upper lip', who manage to put a 'brave face on things'.

This attitude to stress is changing and people are now recognising that we can all have stress, whoever we are.

But stress affects the body. How could that possibly be?

To understand this, let's first talk about Body Language.

Chapter 4
Body Language

Body Language means the variations in posture and appearance that occur naturally and totally without our knowledge or consciousness, as a result of how we feel. The commonest and the easiest to see are the facial expressions (See figure A opposite).

The faces show infinite variations in facial expressions, each showing a different emotion. We can see when people are amused or pleased when their face is smiling; worried or cross when their face is frowning.

The expressions are brought about by the muscles contracting in response to specific emotions. It is an automatic reaction and an accurate reflection of emotion. We do not smile when we are cross and we do not frown when we are pleased.

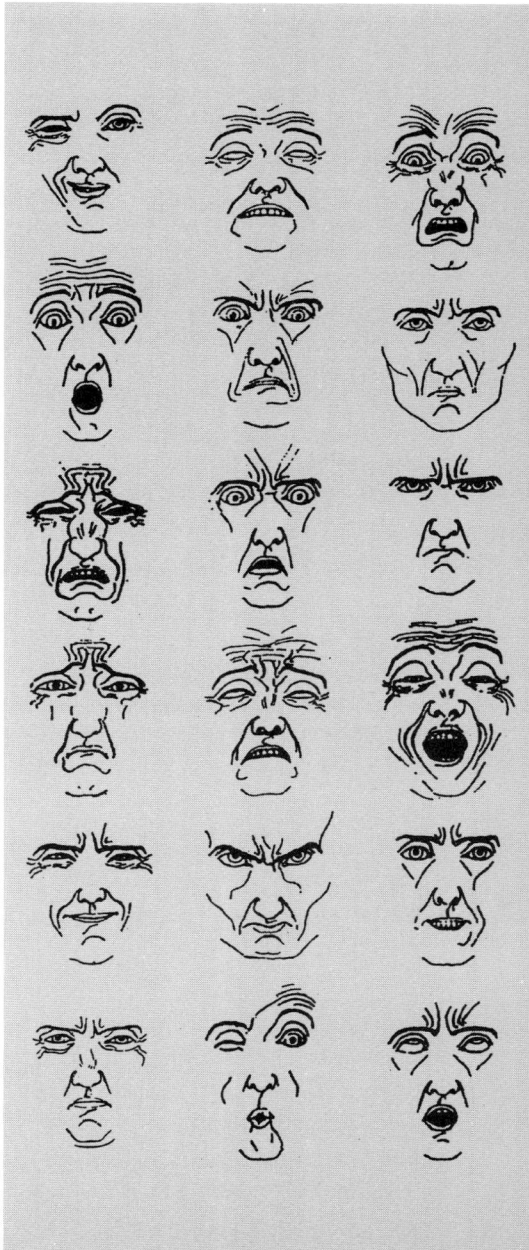

Figure A:
Facial expressions are Body Language at its most obvious. Specific muscles tense in response to specific emotions. It is natural and occurs spontaneously.

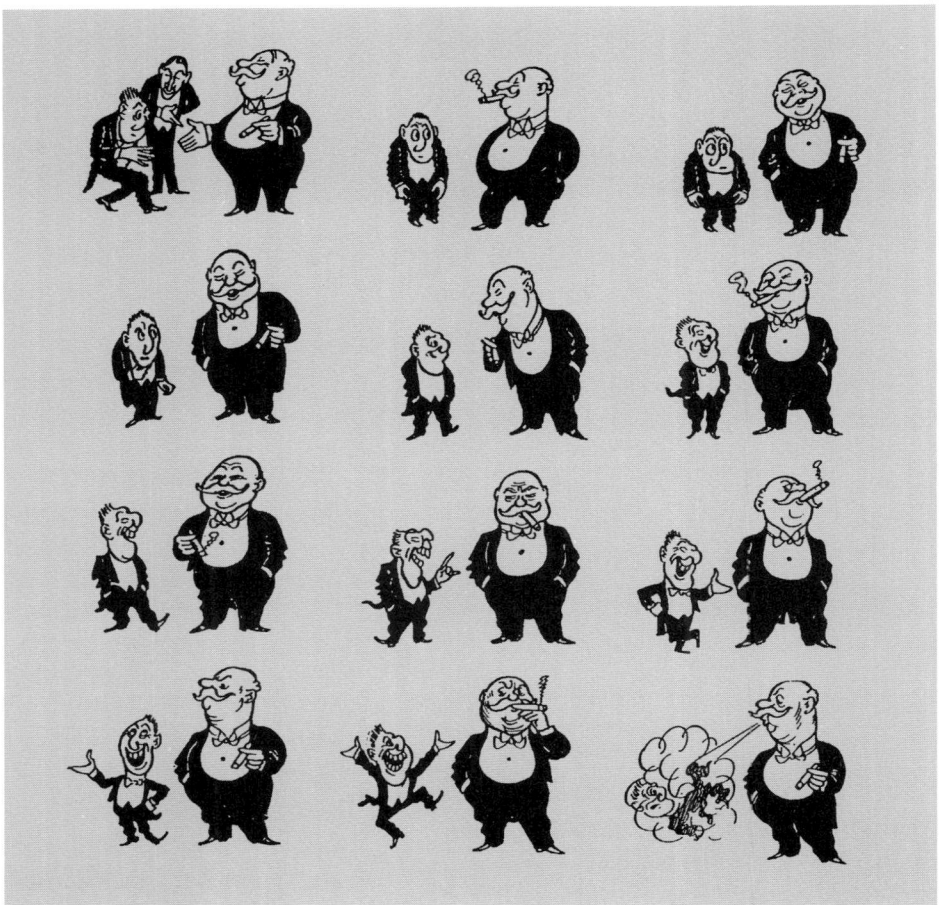

Figure B(i): Body Language. In this cartoon by Bateman, not a word is spoken and yet, by looking at the posture of the two men, we know exactly their emotions. ('Familiarity breeds contempt' © Copyright H.M. Bateman 1969)

This same principle applies to other parts of the body (See figure B(i)).

If you look at Bateman's cartoon, you can tell exactly what the little man's emotions are. He is cowering and his body is slouched (frame one to three) when introduced to the big man who is pompous and intimidating. Gradually the little man achieves success with his conversation, becomes assertive and holds his chin up (frame six), which is all too much for the big man who then puts him down in an aggressive way (frame twelve).

We understand this, not by words, but by the mens' body movements, ie their Body Language. The two mens' movements are natural and not conscious. Their emotions are reflected in their posture. The variation in posture is brought about by the different muscles, to a greater or lesser degree, tensing, or to use another word, contracting.

If the emotions, through Body Language, make our muscles tense, what is it that affects the emotions? The answer is stress. Stress affects our emotions, which affects our Body Language, which makes our muscles tense and keeps them tense. Muscles **which remain tense**, *become painful. So now we know how stress causes muscle pain.*

Chapter 5
Stress – emotions – body language – muscles tense for an extended period – pain

Up to now, although we did not understand how stress could cause pain, we did, nevertheless, often see it in our friends. We saw that they were in pain; we knew that they were going through a stressful time, and we noticed how the pain cleared up when the stress was over.

Although we could see stress and pain in our friends, we did not make the direct link and we certainly did not acknowledge that it might affect ourselves. In fact, if anyone says that our pain is due to stress, we go so far as to take it as an insult, as a criticism of our own ability to cope with life. It is taken as a hurtful criticism because we do not understand the link. The resentment is due to the thought that any pain, due to stress, is 'put on', is 'made up', is even a deliberate attempt to gain sympathy and that it is somehow controlled by the person who is suffering, and that is why we resent it.

It is strange that there is this deep seated resentment to the principle that stress can cause pain, that it can cause any physical reaction in the body, because we frequently see a common occurrence of stress affecting the body. That is blushing. Blushing is a physical reaction to self consciousness, shyness, embarrassment, ie. stress. Sometimes shyness may even lead us to bowing our heads, withdrawing etc. A clear example of body language.

Stress leading to muscle pain can affect all types of people, – business executives, labourers, sedentary workers, housewives, typists, artists and physiotherapists. They are normal, calm, capable people and, as you will see later, it is precisely because they are calm and capable, that they may suffer.

The important point at this stage, is to emphasise very strongly that muscular pain, which results from stress, is *not* put on, it is *not* made up; it is the result of tension in the muscles caused by the reflex of Body Language which occurs outside our control.

So we can now accept that stress, through Body Language, leads to muscular pain.

However, you could say that we all have stress of some sort, at some time or other, but we don't all suffer from muscular pain. No thank goodness, we don't! So why do some people suffer muscular pain and others not? Why does one person suffer sometimes, and not at other times?

The answer is that the muscles become painful when the stress lasts for some time, and *importantly, where we do not allow ourselves free expression.* It occurs when people 'bottle up' their feelings. They do not express their feelings because it would not be socially acceptable to say what they really feel.

They do not say what they really feel because it would hurt somebody else. For example, the mother does not tell her son that his new fiancee is not good enough for him, because she might upset him and lose his affection.

They do not say what they really feel because it might not be in their interest so to do. For example, the new non-smoking office probationer does not complain about their chain smoking boss, because they want to keep their job.

So we now know *how* stress causes pain. What we don't know is why the pain is sometimes in the back and why it is sometimes in the neck.

Why is the pain sometimes in the back and sometimes in the neck?
Well, to understand why the pain is sometimes in the back and sometimes in the neck, we have to look at Body Language. We know that emotion affects Body Language.

So *which* emotion affects the Body Language of the back?
The emotion that affects the Body Language of the back is one where we desparately wish to be dissociated from a situation.

If you look at the little man in Bateman's cartoon, frame 3 (figure B(ii)), you can see his cringing posture. He is cringing because he is

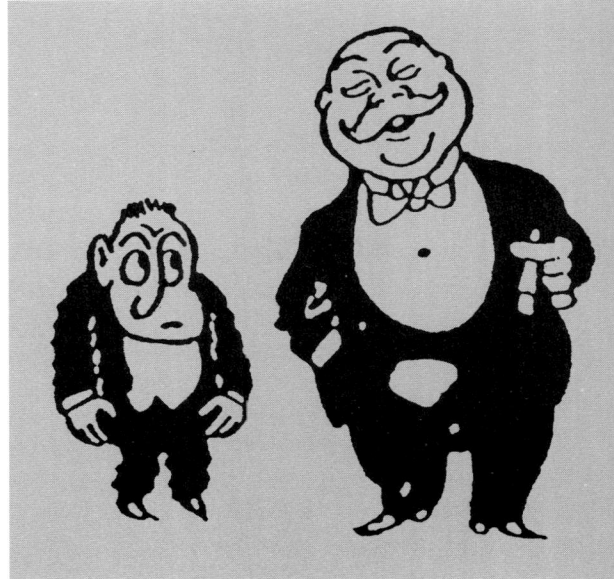

Figure B(ii)

overawed and embarrassed by the overbearing man with the cigar.

His lack of composure is shown in the Body Language of his cringing posture. His cringing posture is brought about by his back and thigh muscles tensing.

We often refer to this Body Language, colloquially, as shrinking from responsibility, cowering with terror or cringing with embarrassment.

If he is very embarrassed, the muscles will be very tense and pull the body out of its usual alignment. If he is not quite so embarrassed, the muscles will be not quite so tense – only a few muscle fibres will be tense, and the posture will look normal.

However, if the emotion persists, especially if we have to 'bottle up' the emotion, the muscles will remain tense. Muscles which *remain tense* become painful.

STRESS – EMOTIONS – BODY LANGUAGE – MUSCLES TENSE FOR AN EXTENDED PERIOD – PAIN

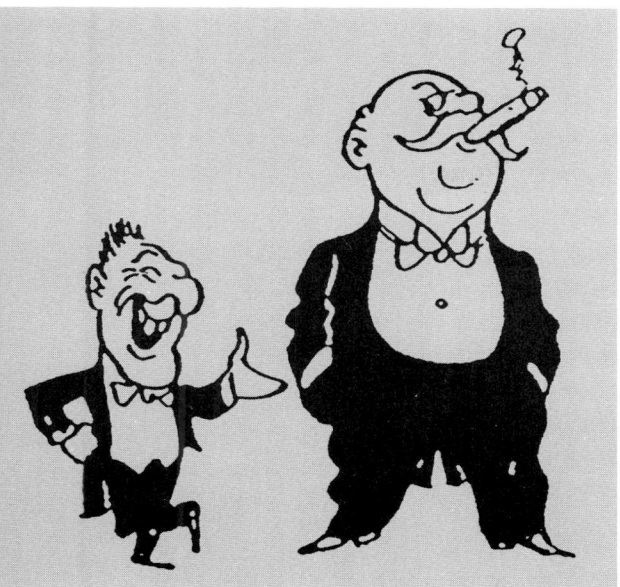

Figure B(iii)

This Body Language in the back is a reflex action and is totally subconscious.

Now to discuss the neck.

So *which* emotion affects the Body Language of the neck?
The emotion that affects the Body Language of the neck is one where we want to be on top of a situation, where we want to be in control.

If you look at the man with the cigar in Bateman's cartoon, frame 9 (figure B(iii)), you can see that he is annoyed with the little man because the little man is taking over the conversation. So the cigar man wants to control him, he wants to squash him. And we can see this by the big man's face and by the tilt backwards of his head – Body Language.

Colloquially, we often refer to this Body Language as "Keep your chin up".

The tilt of the head is brought about by the muscles in the neck. Sometimes they tense so strongly, as in this case, that the neck tilt is visible. Sometimes only a few fibres in the neck muscles tense and the tilt is not visible. However, if the emotion persists, especially if for some reason we have to 'bottle up' our feelings, the muscles will remain tense. Muscles which *remain tense* become painful.

This Body Language in the neck is a reflex action and is totally subconscious.

Chapter 6
Muscles

We know that stress affects the emotions which, through Body Language, make the muscles tense. Some of these specific muscles are referred to later. They stay tense all the time the emotions are affected. Sometimes, although the muscle is painful, it is only a part of a muscle which is tense and the muscle looks normal to the naked eye.

A muscle is composed of many fibres. These fibres can tense or contract a few at a time.

If the emotions are very strong, the muscle is very tense, all the fibres have contracted and it may feel hard. It may be so tense as to pull the body over, – Body Language again. (See figure C).

Look how the head has been tilted backwards and to his left side. The muscles causing this are his left Rectus Capitis Posterior Major and Minor muscles. See later.

Another example is figure D.

Look how the spine is twisted; how the shoulders are not level, the left shoulder is lower than the right shoulder; how the left arm hangs away from the body, – the gap between the trunk and the left arm is wider than the gap on the right side. The muscle causing this incorrect posture is her left Quadratus Lumborum muscle. See later.

If the muscles being used are very tense, they cannot be further used without additional pain. You see this very clearly when you already have backache and you try to bend down to put on your socks or tights. Because of the pain, you cannot reach your feet! Now try to get up. It gets even worse!

Figure C: *Head tipped back by Rectus Capitis Posterior Major and Minor muscles.*

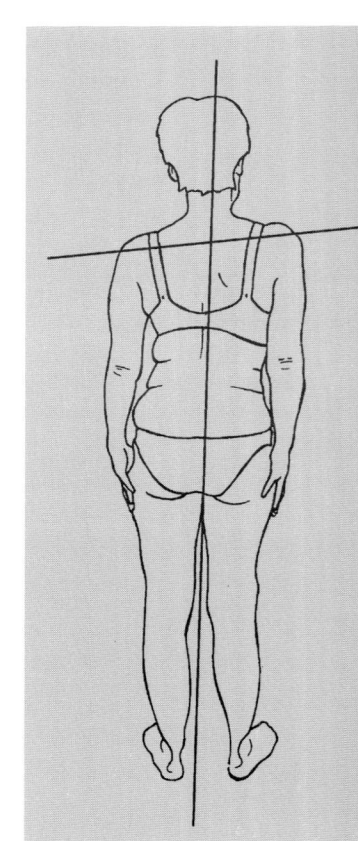

Figure D: *Spine twisted over by Quadratus Lumborum muscle*

Chapter 7
Referred Pain

When these tense and painful muscles become even more tense and painful, as they do when we bend down towards our feet, it is very frightening and the body stiffens even more. It stiffens because other muscles tense to protect the painful area by trying to take some of the load. This second group of muscles which tense, if they remain tense, become painful. They may be near the original pain, or further away, such as in the arm or down the leg. And so you have a spread of pain. This spread of pain is called REFERRED PAIN.

There is referred pain also, when muscles tense in order to protect an injury, but we are not discussing injuries in this book.

Which muscles are they that can give rise to referred pain? They are numerous and varied; they can be very painful and they need treatment. However, when the main muscle problem is treated and cured, the referred pain will naturally settle down.

Chapter 8
Changes in Pain

Why does the pain move sometimes?
The pain might move from one place to another because we have changed our attitude to the original stress. The original stress still bothers us, but instead of wanting nothing to do with it, we have now decided to deal with it positively. As soon as we decide this, the pain moves from the back to the neck!

Oh dear, but it might happen!

Why does it happen? It happens because we are still in a stressful situation. But it is one we are handling differently and which, therefore, affects us differently. When we finally deal with the entire circumstance giving rise to the original stress to our satisfaction, all our pain is finally cleared.

Why does the pain fluctuate sometimes?
IT COMES AND GOES. One of the most noticeable and baffling aspects of this complaint is how the pain 'comes and goes'. It comes and goes without any apparent reason. Why?

We have established that the muscles can tense and become painful due to stress. However, stress fluctuates. We have a problem which is 'needling' us and about which we have to bottle up our feelings. Sometimes this is at the forefront of our minds, and we are feeling extremely concerned about it. So the muscle will be extremely tense and therefore extremely painful.

On the other hand, we may be busy and thinking of something else, so the stress is at the back of our minds. We are not, at that moment, feeling quite so strongly about it, the muscles are not so tense and, therefore, not so painful.

This shows how pain comes and goes.

Anxiety
Anxiety is common in neck pain and backache, —anxiety about the cause of pain. When the pain 'just comes on', we look for an accident, some physical strains at work or home. When there has been none, and before we go to the doctor, we are naturally concerned and worry. The commonest worry is that we have cancer. This worry, however, increases the muscle tension and so increases the pain. When we realise we do not have a disease or illness, the pain eases.

This further shows how the pain comes and goes.

Chapter 9
Pain and the Nerve Receptors

We need to understand a little about the anatomy of muscles. Normal muscle contraction, as when walking across a room, or with any normal movement, is not painful.

The muscles, however, do become painful when there is excessive contraction, as in cramp, or excessive contraction due to tension of part of a muscle. This can be confined to a few muscle fibres only, or a few motor units as they are called, as occurs in common neck and back ache. This type of pain is of an aching quality, and may be stabbing, shooting, gripping or nagging.

When a tense muscle is made even more tense (by giving it resistance so that it has to tense harder), the muscle becomes much more painful. When the same muscle is relaxed, the pain is reduced to the original level. To make sure that the extra pain is coming from the muscle and not from the underlying joint, the joint is kept still when resistance is given to the muscle. When the muscle is totally relaxed the pain goes.

In these tense and painful muscles there are spots which are even more painful. They are called 'trigger spots'. These trigger spots are always found in the same place, at either end of the muscle, at the point where the muscle is attached to the bone.

Pressure on a trigger spot elicits severe and agonising pain. These trigger spots are found only in a tense aching muscle and disappear with improvement of the condition. The trigger spots are found in exactly the same part of a muscle as the specialised part of a nerve, ie. a 'nerve ending'. The specialised nerve endings, or receptors, at the ends of muscles are called Golgi tendon organs.

In the group of nerve receptors, Golgi tendon organs are one of the nerve receptors for feelings of movement. They are termed one of the kinaesthetic receptors.

The kinaesthetic receptors tell us what position our bodies are in, even when our eyes are closed. For instance, if we close our eyes, stretch our arms to the ceiling, and keep our eyes closed, it is the kinaesthetic receptors which tell us that our arms are up there and that they have not dropped down. If we keep our eyes closed and slowly lower our arms so that they are stretched out sideways like an aeroplane, it is the kinaesthetic receptors which tell us where our arms are in relationship to our body.

It maybe that the Golgi tendon organs play a double role. They are the nerve receptors for feelings of movement. However, when they are overstimulated as in continuous muscle tension due to stress, they become painful.

Thus as well as being the nerve receptors for feelings of movement, Golgi tendon organs are also the nerve receptors for aching pain.

Chapter 10
Treatment to Necks and Backs

Although the pain we are discussing is fundamentally due to stress, the reaction in the body of the muscles contracting and being tense is a physical one, and it is physical treatment that is necessary to alleviate the pain, whether the treatment is done by the patient at home, or whether the patient seeks treatment from a physiotherapist.

The aim of the treatment is to relax the muscle and, if possible, address the cause – the stress. The muscle problem and the stress cause are inextricably linked and should both be addressed at the same time. Because one is physical treatment and the other is treatment by counselling, they are described separately. A trained physiotherapist would handle both aspects of the treatment at the same time.

However, patients may well find that they can treat themselves. They can treat the muscles by following the specific advice given, as far as they are able, or by adapting it to their own convenience. They can treat the stress by recognising problems, talking them over with trusted colleagues, and taking action to overcome the problem if this is possible. In many instances this is not possible by self counselling and advice of a trained counsellor should be sought.

Treatment of the muscle by the patient

Physical relaxation of the muscle and the easing of pain is obtained by:

a) Heat; either a hot water bottle, hot baths, hot packs or a heat lamp. Heat is necessary for the following reasons:

   i) Heat brings more blood to the muscles. The oxygen in the blood neutralises the excess lactic acid that has built up as a result of the muscle tension. Over-used muscle makes excess lactic acid and excess lactic acid makes the muscle slightly short and prevents it from returning to its original length. This is important to realise because the patient may already have learnt the art of relaxation and be good at it, but if there is excess lactic acid, the muscle will remain in a shortened state and therefore not be relaxed.

   ii) Heat helps to relax the muscle. Just as heat makes the majority of matter extend, it makes the muscle extend. The heat should be appreciably warm, but don't, obviously, burn yourself.

b) Massage of the muscle (see chapter 22) can be a help and can be from a willing relative, or from a professional therapist.

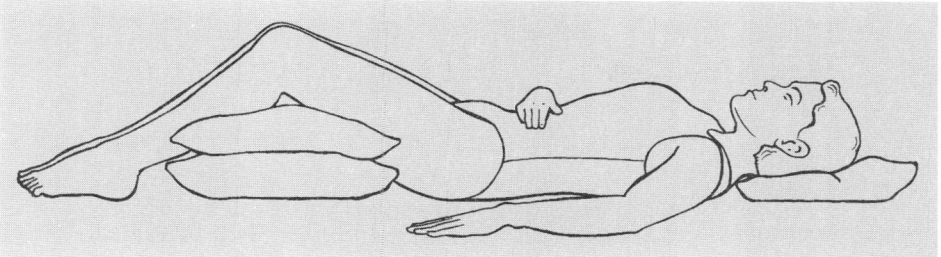

*Figure E: Breathing for relaxation. When relaxing, breathe with the diaphragm. Place one hand on the abdomen; as you breathe in the abdomen goes up, as you breathe out, it sinks down towards the bed. Breathe slowly, rhythmically, **not deeply**. Think about the breathing.*

c) Relaxation of the muscle by the patient.
Some people say they do not know whether they are relaxed or not. So, to learn relaxation of one muscle, it is necessary to learn how to relax all muscles. To do this the body needs to be comfortably supported and warm. The aim is to let the trunk and limbs feel heavy and lifeless, the same feeling you get immediately before you drop off to sleep, or when you feel too lazy to be bothered doing anything.

To help achieve this, try slow breathing with the diaphragm. Lie down, place one hand on the abdomen, as in figure E. Breathe in and the abdomen comes up towards the ceiling, breathe out and it sinks back down towards the floor.

Breathe slowly, not too deeply, a gentle breath in, a gentle breath out. Big deep breaths are not necessary, and they only make us hyperventilate. This is unpleasant and does not help relaxation.

The rhythm of the breathing is helped by silently saying one's name to oneself, eg. Jenny. JEN as you breathe in, NEE as you breathe out. This technique is simple but it is very effective in creating a steady rhythm.

The even rhythm of breathing is good for two reasons:

i) It stops us holding our breath. Pain makes us hold our breath, or breathe irregularly and in a shallow manner, which prevents relaxation. With intense pain, the condition is much more severe and it makes the muscles more tense, and so increases the pain;

ii) It gives us something to think about, so that we are not thinking about the stress, and this, though minor, can be very effective.

It is no use saying don't think about your problems. You can say don't move your arm and you don't, but when you say don't think about your problems, you find that 'the mind has escaped' and the problem is exactly what you are thinking about! So try

BAD BACKS AND PAINFUL PARTS

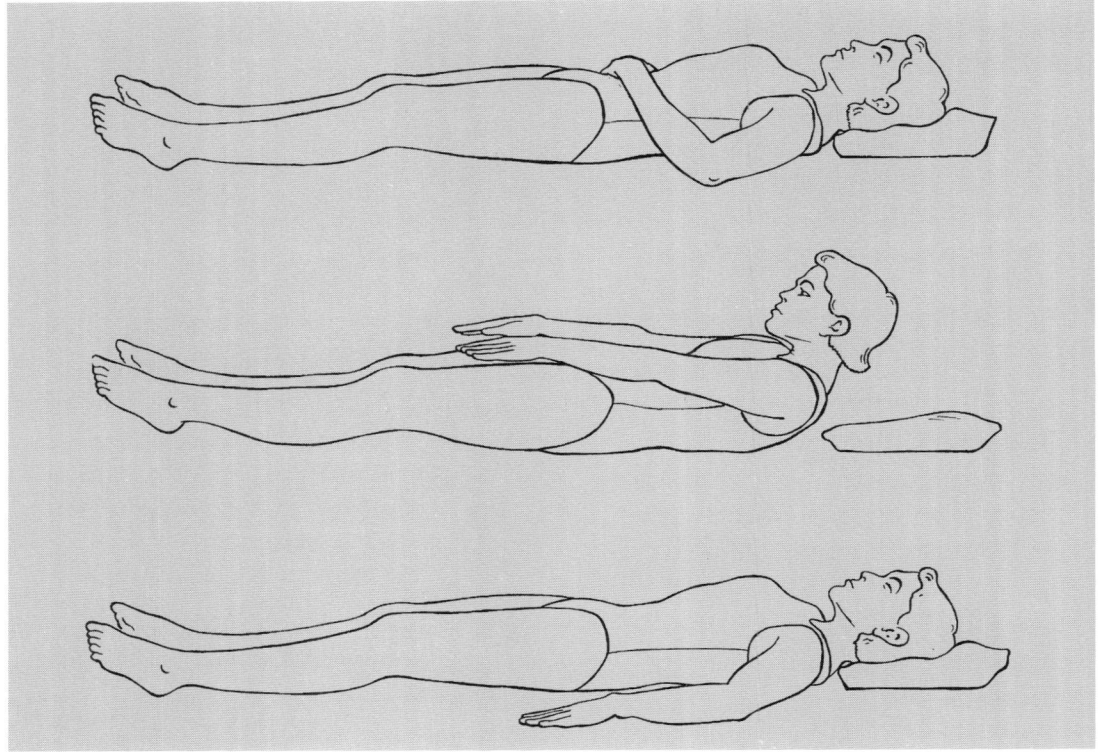

Figures F: (i, ii and iii). Testing yourself for relaxation

concentrating on something positive, such as the breathing.

Questionable technique

For relaxation some use the technique of tightening everything up and then letting go, but although it is easy to tighten up, it is very difficult to let go. After all, when you have tightened up, you then have to let go down to a level beyond where you were already. So why bother tightening up, – it is not logical.

Testing yourself for relaxation

The preferred technique is to lie down with a supportive pillow, let the limbs feel heavy and lifeless and practise the diaphragmatic breathing (Fi). Then point your toes, brace your knees, lift your head in order to look towards your toes. Count 10 (Fii). Then 'collapse' back into relaxation (Fiii). The arms and legs feel floppy and lifeless and you breathe slowly with the diaphragm.

Treatment of the muscle by a Chartered Physiotherapist

The body is not good at localising pain and the patient is often quite vague when trying to pin point it. If the pain is very severe, a Chartered Physiotherapist can localise the exact muscles. The more intense the pain, the easier it is to pinpoint the muscles.

As the pain reduces it is harder to pinpoint. A therapist, who specialises in massaging and manipulating muscles, providing 'hands on' treatment, may be needed for relaxing them.

Relaxation involves passively moving various parts of the body in a slow, rhythmical and repetitive way. It is repeated until the muscles are relaxed. There should not be any forced or jerking movements. At the same time, the patient lets the arms and legs, and even the head, go totally limp.

The therapist uses the method as a means of testing, to ascertain if the muscles are totally relaxed. However, it can also be used to teach the patient to relax. By the physiotherapist continuing to carry out the passive movements, the patient is able to practise relaxing the muscles.

So it is a testing and a teaching process of relaxation.

Passive movement also helps improve the blood supply, which, as previously stated, brings more oxygen to the muscles to neutralise excess lactic acid and so help the muscle to attain its original length.

There are additional treatments, such as pain killers or electrical therapy, which may be provided by a doctor, chemist, or chartered physiotherapist. However, the aim of this book is to explain to patients, how they may handle, and treat, the complaint by themselves.

Newspapers and magazines tend, these days, to suggest that we must all be relaxed all of the time. This is wrong. If we were totally relaxed all of the time, we would be like cabbages.

The opposite of relaxation is tension. To be tense means to be alert, to be ready for action. We will never get anything done unless we are tense or alert. The only trouble with tension is that, in the case of muscles when they are too tense for too long, they become painful. Remember, it has already been explained that when a muscle, or a few fibres in a muscle, *remain tense*, they become painful.

People should learn the art of relaxation so that when they have the need to use it, they know what to do. They should learn to 'melt the pain away' by relaxing, rather than trying to 'fight the pain away' by remaining tense.

Chapter 11
Treatment of stress
How to get rid of the cause
– the stress itself

It is true that some people are not interested in the cause. They are content with self help, or professional therapy, on the muscles only. That is perfectly acceptable, so long as they will accept the principle of stress causing pain and that they must have something stressful affecting them.

For those who want to know the cause of the pain, some thought may be given as to a possible stress causing the tension. They should recall how they felt when the pain first came on, and what they were thinking about at the time, so that they understand for themselves, the cause and effect. Sometimes this is crystal clear to someone suffering muscular pain due to stress, eg. the pain came on some time after they were told they might be made redundant. If they want to discuss the stress with their physiotherapist, they will be given kindness, understanding and, of course, privacy.

Sometimes the cause is not so clear, and the link may not be seen. In this event it may be necessary to seek help from a professional counsellor, in order to recall the situation that is relevant. The counselling process can in itself give relief, because relaxation may be temporarily induced.

Some people may not want to talk to their therapist, they may prefer to talk to their best friend, their best relative, or a complete stranger. Talking to a supportive friend, or relative, is counselling. Counselling is fully recognised now as being a powerful tool in dealing with personal stressful problems. Some may not wish to talk at all and prefer to deal with a stress inducing problem themselves. This can be appropriate but it may well be harder to do.

Having realised for themselves what the stress is, the patient has either to remove it, or change their attitude towards it, so that it is no longer stressful. If both of these are impossible and they may well be, they should try to forget it, even if only for a short time. Then they should relax, follow the self help treatment to ease the pain, and so get on with life.

Chapter 12
Summary

Stress affects the emotions, which affects Body Language, which affects the muscles.

1) As a reaction to stress or to a 'problem' in life, the muscles in the body tense. Sometimes this is visible and is called Body Language. Sometimes only part of a muscle tenses and it is not visible.

2) This is a normal reaction, it is a reflex and is totally subconscious.

3) The muscles that tense depend on the person's reaction to the stress. Different reactions bring about different Body Language. Different Body Language uses different muscles.

4) If the reaction to the stress is to want to master the situation, or to want to get on top of it, or to want to overcome some failure, the Body Language will affect the neck muscles. In life, the Body Language in the neck is often seen and described colloquially as "Keeping your chin up", or "Holding your head high".

5) If the reaction to the stress is to want to shrink away from it, to want to have nothing to do with it, the Body Language will affect the muscles in the back. The Body Language seen in the back is often referred to as cringing.

Colloquially, when talking of an unbearable situation, we use the phrase, "I cringe when I think of it".

6) Tense muscles which *remain tense, become painful.*

7) Treatment is aimed at relaxation of these muscles and, if necessary, addressing the cause.

Chapter 13
Support for the Neck and the Back

Always try to support areas when lying or sitting, to ease the pain and promote relaxation. If the pain is severe, the body must be given support. The following are simple, practical methods for you to use and help yourself.

In bed with neck pain
There are many proprietary brands of mechanical support on the market. However, you can also make your own (McKenzie, Robin. *See* Bibliography).

A towel is rolled into a long 'sausage', using two elastic bands. Figure G(i). This sausage, called a cervical roll, is then placed inside the pillow case. Figure G(ii).

Figure G(i), (ii), (iii):
Support for the neck

This cervical roll gives support to the neck and is comfortable when lying on your back or on your side. Figure G(iii).

In bed with backache
a) Put two really fat pillows, or cushions, under the knees. Figure H.

These take the strain off the back. It has the added advantage that because the hips and knees are bent in the same way as when you are lying on your side, you do not have the normal urge to turn onto your side which is an extremely painful, if not impossible action, when you have a bad back.

b) If you need to sleep on your side, put two really fat pillows between the knees so that the top knee is on the

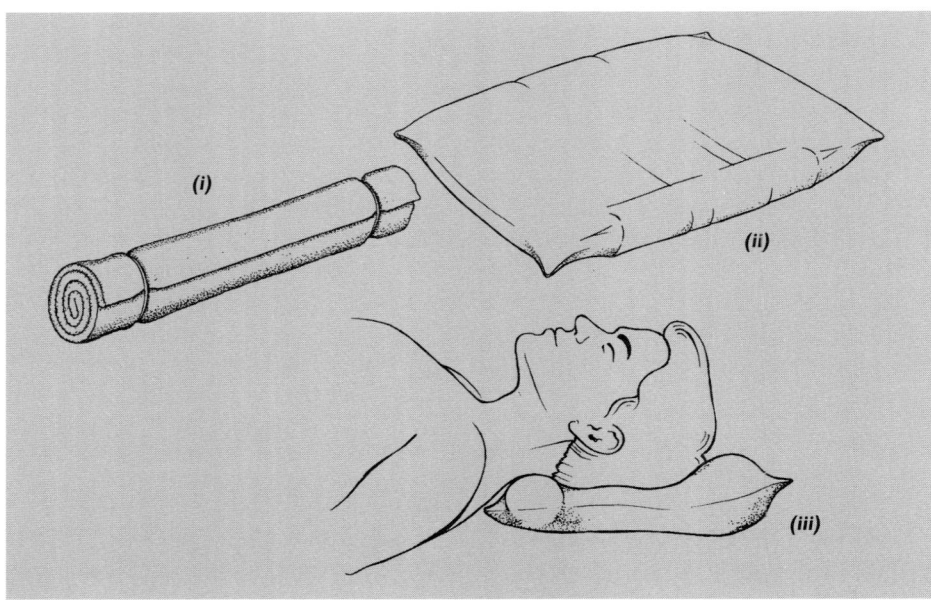

SUPPORT FOR THE NECK AND THE BACK

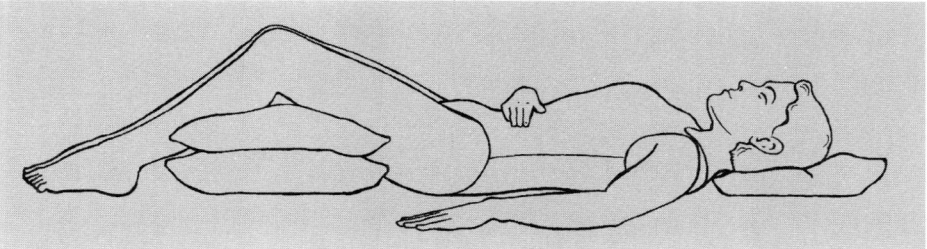

Figure H: Support for the back

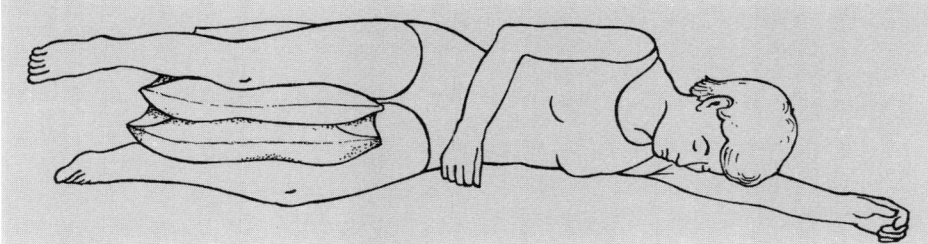

Figure I: Support for the back when lying on your side

same level as the hip. Figure I. This prevents a drag on the back. The underneath arm does not need to be outstretched as in the picture; put it wherever it is most comfortable.

Sitting on a chair with backache

Figure J(i) shows the wrong way to sit on a chair, whilst figure J(ii) shows the correct way to sit on a chair, that is, with support for the natural curve in you back.

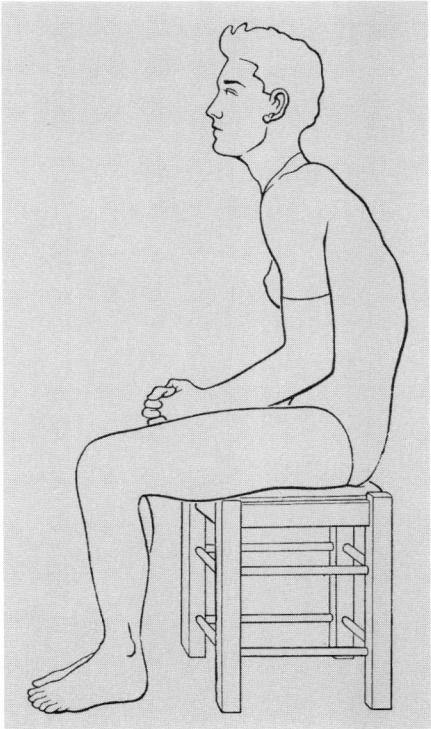

Figure J(i): Wrong way to sit on a chair

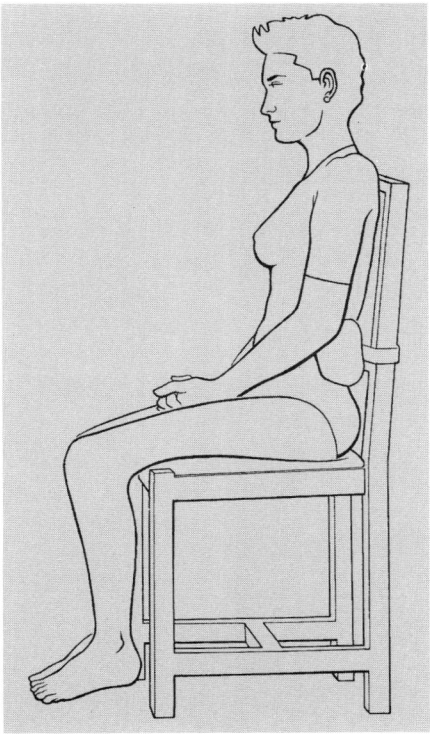

Figure J(ii): Right way to sit on a chair

You will see that there is a small cushion in the 'small' of your back. This is called a lumbar roll.

When sitting, sit back on the seat, place the lumbar roll behind the back, about waist level. The roll maintains the natural curve of the back passively, so that you can then relax. It is wrong to try to keep the natural curve of the back by using your muscles. This only increases the muscle tension, and so increases the pain. So use the lumbar roll, and relax as best you can.

Lumbar Rolls

There are many proprietary brands on the market which can be strapped to the chair, figure K(i).

However, you can also make your own.

D.I.Y. Lumbar Roll

This is easy to make. Roll a towel and secure it into shape using a needle and thread, or, easier still, use two elastic bands. Figure K(ii).

Alternatively, you can use the modern packaging material, bubble wrap. Make a roll and secure it with the two elastic bands.

Use the roll at the office, at home or when driving the car.

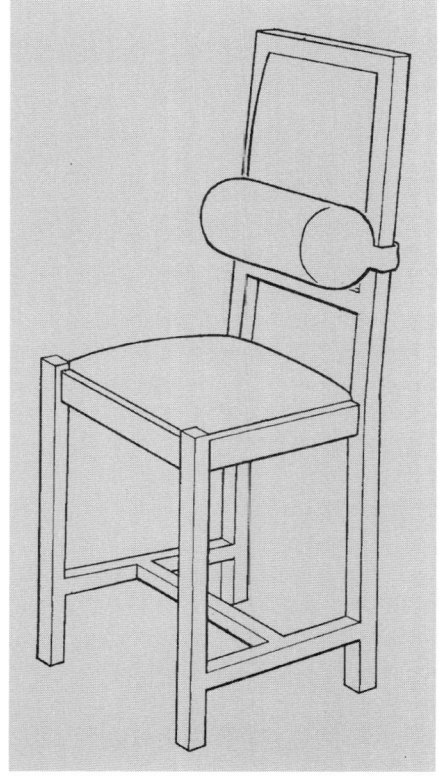

Figure K(i): *Support for the back*

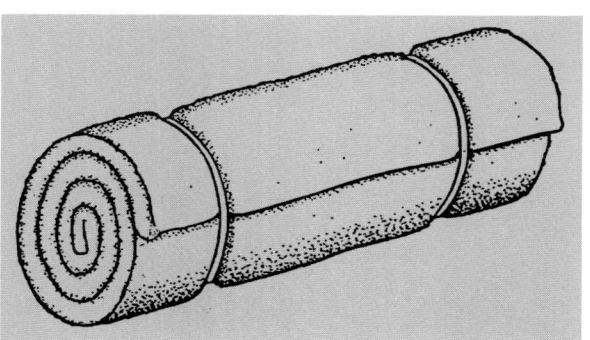

Figure K(ii):
DIY support for the back

Chapter 14
Examples of Stress and the Main Muscles involved

I hesitate to give examples because when people find that they do not apply to themselves, they tend to reject the whole concept. It cannot be emphasised too strongly that there are an infinite number of stressful situations, and moreover, what is a stress to one, would leave another unmoved. There is no right and wrong type of stress. Stress is individually determined and it is only what that person concerned thinks, that matters.

Muscles are given names in Latin. The fact that small muscles can have long names, does not make them user-friendly! However, don't let that put you off. This book will show you pictures of the muscles so that you can locate them approximately yourself. Accurate location can be achieved by a physiotherapist. The book will help you to understand what the muscles do and why they become painful and this will help you to ease and then get rid of the pain. That is what matters.

Examples of stress affecting the neck
The examples are, of course, suitably disguised.

1) A new supervisor wanted to totally reorganise his office but to do so, needed the co-operation of the staff. The staff, though pleasant and hard working were unwilling to make any changes. The supervisor did not want to upset them and the nice atmosphere in the office, but was determined to bring about the changes and as a result, developed pain in the neck with headaches as well. These headaches are muscular pain also. The pain lasted on and off for several weeks until he finally got the office to his liking.

The muscles involved were RECTUS CAPITIS POSTERIOR MAJOR and MINOR and OCCIPITO FRONTALIS.

2) A shy old lady, who lived on her own, complained to the neighbours of the loud music and late party noise, but they took no notice. She wanted to ask again but was too shy. But she did really want the noise to stop and developed pain in the neck. Suddenly, and unexpectedly, the neighbours moved. Wonderful! The lady's neck improved immediately.

The muscle involved was LEVATOR SCAPULAE.

3) A forty year old lady took her driving test and failed. She took it twice more but unfortunately, she failed again. She developed pain in her neck as she desperately wanted to drive but was not allowed to as she had not passed her test and she felt her age was against her also.

The muscle involved was LEVATOR SCAPULAE.

Examples of stress affecting the back
The examples are suitably disguised.

1) A lady went to visit her favourite brother who was in hospital. He told her that he was diagnosed as having a terminal illness. To her brother she was supportive, but she could not bear to think of losing him and developed acute pain in the back.

The muscles involved were QUADRATUS LUMBORUM and TENSOR FASCIAE LATAE.

2) A middle aged man, "a pillar of the community", was due to appear in court charged with shop lifting. He dreaded it; he wanted to run away. Before he appeared, he developed acute back pain and sciatica spreading into the lower leg.

The muscles involved were the HAMSTRINGS and SOLEUS.

3) A widower, who lived on his own, mixed with other people at work during the week, but at weekends he was on his own and loathed it. During the week he had no pain, but every weekend when feeling lonely, he had pain down the outside of the upper leg.

The muscle involved was TENSOR FASCIAE LATAE.

4) A man had severe backache and sciatica when his wife was having a 'secret' affair. Everyone knew, they were laughing at him and the husband could not bear it.

The muscles involved were QUADRATUS LUMBORUM and the HAMSTRINGS.

5) A lady had put her son through university and he had gained a good degree. However, he could not get a job. He filled his time labouring and when he was again turned down for an appropriate job which used his degree, his mother was upset. She could not bear to think of him being prevented from using his education and she developed backache.

The muscle involved was QUADRATUS LUMBORUM.

As you can see, the stress may be at home with one's family, friends or neighbours; it may be at work with one's superiors, peers or subordinates; it may concern acquaintances in clubs, politics or hobbies. The variety is infinite.

Chapter 15
Muscles involved

The muscles involved in stress related pain are the prime movers. They are the main muscles which produce a specific movement, and they lie mostly in the deeper layers of the muscles.

Those in the neck area are:
RECTUS CAPITIS POSTERIOR MAJOR and MINOR (Figure L).

LEVATOR SCAPULAE (Figure L)

Those on the scalp are:
OCCIPITO FRONTALIS and AURICULARES (Figures M(i) and (ii)).

Those in the back and the back and side of the leg are:
QUADRATUS LUMBORUM. (Figure N)
TENSOR FASCIAE LATAE. (Figure O)
HAMSTRINGS. (Figure P)
SOLEUS (Figure Q)

The muscles involved in referred pain are numerous and varied.

Referred pain in the neck area might involve Occipito frontalis, Deltoid, Supraspinatus, Extensors of the wrist, Pectoralis major or Rhomboids.

Referred pain in the back area might involve Iliocostalis, External rotators of the hip, Psoas and Iliacus, Rectus abdominis, Hamstrings, Soleus, Tibialis posterior or Serratus anterior.

Don't worry about these names, but those who do know their muscles can see that there can be quite a spread and quite a number of them. Each can be separately located by a physiotherapist and treated accordingly.

The muscles involved in stress related pain are pictured and described separately on the following pages, together with hints on how to deal with the problem and simple exercises are given. *Remember*, after every exercise, always move in as relaxed a way as possible. Try not to hold yourself tense. Don't hold your breath. Breathe with your diaphragm (tummy muscles) slowly, rhythmically and not too deeply.

The muscles of the neck – Rectus Capitis Posterior Major and Minor (Figure L)

Main actions: These two muscles tip the head backwards and turn it to the same side as the muscle is on.

Painful everyday actions and how to minimise them:

1) Looking up at the ceiling – postpone papering the ceiling!

2) Bending forward as in computer keyboard work or reading a book on your lap – raise your typewriter, computer keyboard or book, to a more comfortable level.

3) Knitting – don't knit meantime.

4) Washing your hair in the wash basin – wash your hair while standing in the shower.

5) Turning your head when reversing the car – drive the car making full use of the mirrors.

6) Swimming breast stroke with your head out of the water – change from breast stroke to back stroke, or, if you don't want to get your hair wet, try side stroke.

Simple exercise, preferably after heat:

a) Firstly, turn your head gently, *away* from the pain. If the pain is on both sides, turn your head away from the most painful side first. So if the pain is on your left side, turn your head to the right. Stop when it hurts, turn the face to the front again. Repeat this, gently increasing the range, millimetre by millimetre.

b) Secondly, turn gently into the pain. DON'T force it. Just do it bit by bit. Repeat several times.

When exercising, don't bother moving your head up and down. However bad the pain, you will do a little bit of this movement naturally as you go about your life. Do not do circular rolling movements of the head, as this does not give a full range of movement and it might make you dizzy. Furthermore, it tends to make the neck 'creak'. The creaking is the cartilage (gristle) rubbing on itself and although this does not matter, people do not like the noise, and it doesn't help anyway.

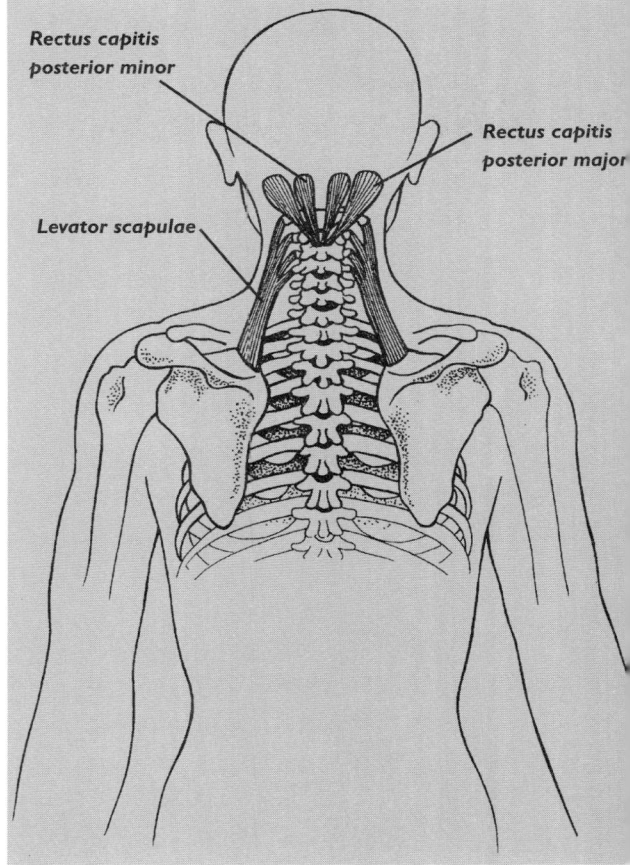

Figure L: *Muscles of the neck*

Don't tip your head back so your chin is in the air, but do tuck your chin down so that you form a long neck at the back.

When in bed, make sure you are not pressing your head into the pillow and sticking your chin up. Instead, bring your chin down and again form a long neck at the back.

MUSCLES INVOLVED

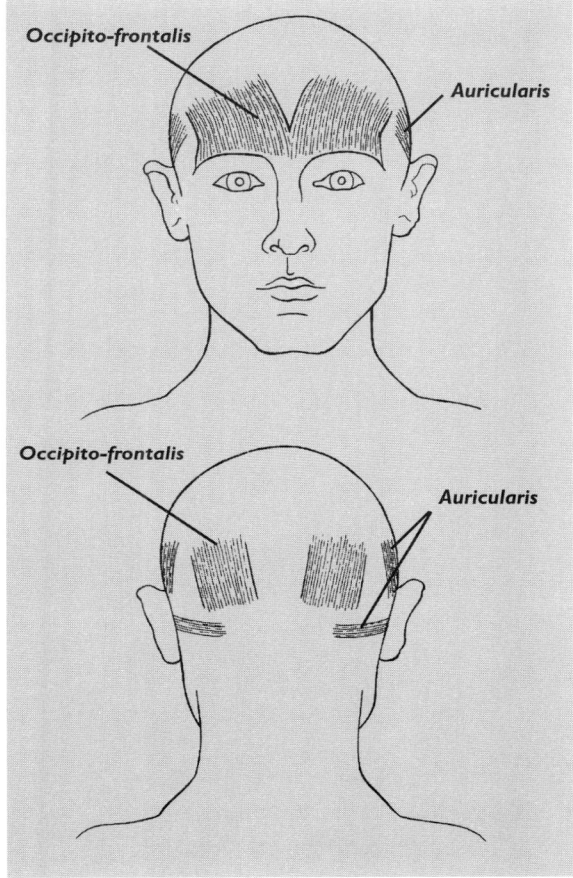

Figures M(i) and (ii): Muscles of the scalp

The muscle of the neck – Levator Scapulae (Figure L)

Main action: This muscle raises the shoulder blade.

Painful everyday actions and how to minimise pain:

1) Carrying a heavy shoulder bag, or heavy shopping, on the painful side – carry your shoulder bag, or your shopping, on your other arm.

2) Driving with hunched shoulders – when driving, sit back in your seat and drop your shoulders.

3) Generally having hunched shoulders – look at your reflection in a mirror, or shop window, to see if your shoulders are hunched. If they are, drop them!

4) When using the telephone, don't clamp it between your ear and shoulder – hold the phone in your hand.

Simple exercise, preferably after heat:

Shrug your shoulders up and down several times, making sure that you finish with them down.

The muscles of the scalp – Occipito-frontalis and Auriculares (Figures M (i and ii))

Main actions: These muscles raise our eyebrows and waggle our ears.

To minimise pain: Massage the scalp, ie. make circular and stroking movements across the forehead, and circular movements on the scalp. It is often particularly painful behind the ears – so painful that we think that we have earache. If you ask your doctor and he says that there is nothing wrong with your ears, then concentrate the massage on the scalp behind the ears.

The muscle of the back – Quadratus Lumborum (Figure N)

Main actions:

1) This muscle and the same muscle on the other side straighten the back up, after stooping forwards.

2) When standing on one leg, the muscle on the opposite side of the body helps to balance the body.

3) The muscle bends the trunk sideways, to the same side as the muscle.

4) When lying down, the muscle and the same muscle on the other side, arches the back.

Painful everyday actions and how to minimise pain:

1) Bending down to lift anything up – don't lift; but if you must, then keep a straight back and bend the knees.

2) Stooping, as when stooping over the lawn mower, or leaning over the basin when cleaning one's teeth – don't stay in the bent position for a long time. Interrupt your bending with standing and arching backwards.

3) Bending down to put on your trousers – when putting on trousers, safety pin a towel on to the waist band, drop the trousers to the floor and pull up on the towel.

4) Standing on one leg in order to put on your sock or stocking – sit down to put on your sock or stocking. If you cannot reach, ask someone to help, even a colleague at work!

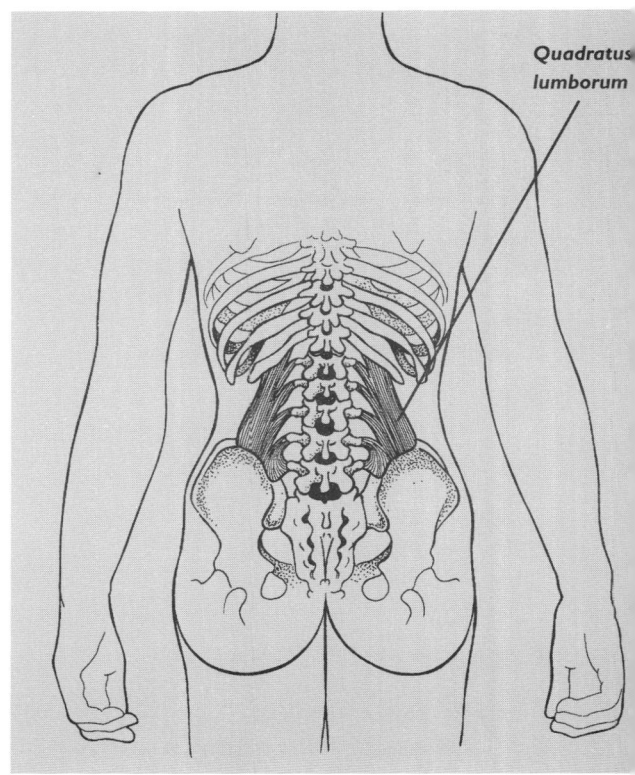

Figure N: *Muscles of the back*

5) Getting in and out of the car, and changing gear whilst driving – wearing a shiny plastic mac helps you slide more easily on your seat to reach the gear lever and when getting in and out of the car.

6) Sitting down and standing up – when sitting down try and use a chair with arms so you can take your weight through your arms. Don't sit for long periods. Get up and move about.

7) Turning over in bed and getting out of bed – when lying on your back, put two fat pillows under your knees. This not only takes the strain off your back, it also saves the need for turning on to your side in order to bend your knees.

When getting out of bed, turn onto your painful side, put your feet over the edge of the bed and sit up sideways. It is then the good side that does the lifting, not the painful side.

Simple exercise, preferably after heat:

a)   Lie on your back, make the leg on the painful side longer, and stretch the arm on the same side up above your head. Relax. Repeat several times.

b)   Lie on your back, bend first one knee up on to your chest and then put it down. Alternate with the other leg. Relax. Repeat several times.

c)   When standing, put your hands in the hollow of your back and arch backwards. Repeat several times.

d)   Relax whenever you can.

Bear in mind that, with Quadratus Lumborum, the pain is often experienced only at the very lowest end of the muscle, where it is attached to the bone but you still have to treat the whole muscle.

The muscle at the side of the thigh – Tensor Fasciae Latae (Figure O)

Main Actions:

1)   When standing on one leg, the muscle balances the body on that leg.

2)   The muscle lifts the leg out to the same side as the muscle and rotates it inwards.

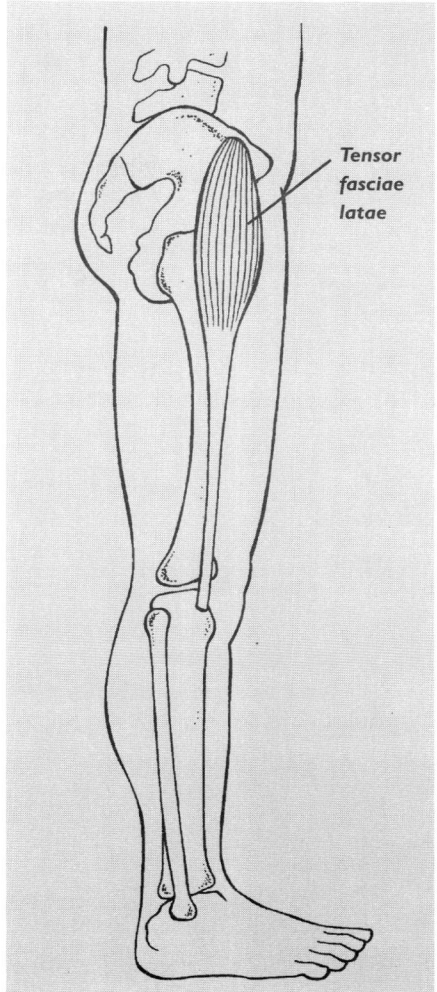

Figure O: *Muscle at the side of the leg*

3)   In the erect position, the muscle steadies the body on top of the legs.

Painful everyday actions and how to minimise pain:

1)   Standing on one leg – stand on both legs with your feet apart. However, walking about is easier than standing still.

2)   Sitting with your legs crossed – don't!

Simple exercise, preferably after heat:

Lie on your back, keep your leg straight. Roll the whole leg out, then roll it in.

Repeat several times, but finish with it rolled out. You can also do this when standing.

With Tensor Fasciae Latae, the patient often experiences pain only in the foreleg, below the knee, ie. where the muscle is attached to the tibia.

However, the whole muscle needs to be treated.

The muscles at the back of the thigh – the Hamstrings
ie. *Semimembranosus, Semitendinosus, Biceps Femoris* (Figure P)

Main Actions:

1) These muscles bend the knee.

2) These muscles prevent the trunk falling forward and help to keep it erect whilst we are standing.

3) When the body is bent forward at the hips, these muscles raise it back to the erect position.

4) These muscles extend the leg backwards.

Painful everyday actions and how to minimise pain:

Some of the following actions are performed by both Quadratus lumborum and the Hamstrings.

1) Bending down and lifting anything up, such as a suitcase – don't lift, but if you must, take some of the

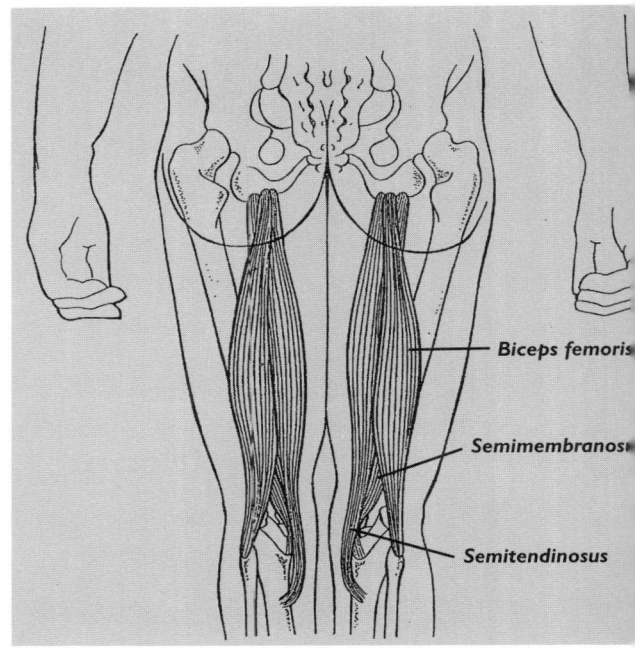

Figure P: *Muscles at the back of thigh*

weight with one hand placed on your thigh, (see figure S(iii)), or put one hand on a chair and take your weight through that.

2) Bending down and then straightening up after having put on your sock or stocking – again take your weight with one hand placed on your thigh, or put one hand on a chair and take your weight through that.

3) Stooping, as when hoovering the carpet or leaning over the wash basin washing your face – don't stoop for long periods. Interrupt it with standing and arching backwards.

4) Standing up and sitting down – when sitting, use only a chair with arms so that you can lower yourself and stand up, by taking the weight through your own arms. Before sitting, stretch the painful leg forwards, and then lower

yourself taking the weight through the 'good' leg. Don't sit for long periods. Get up and move about. Some people like rocking in a rocking chair.

5) Climbing stairs – climb the stairs with the 'good' leg only, and the 'bad' leg follows behind. Each step is climbed with the 'good' leg. Coming down stairs it is the reverse. Every time, the 'bad' leg goes down first.

6) Kneeling on one knee – if you must kneel, then only kneel down on the knee which is on the same side as the pain.

7) Getting in and out of the car and changing gear whilst driving – wearing a shiny plastic mac helps you slide more easily on your seat when changing gear and when getting in and out of the car.

8) Turning over in bed – when lying in bed on your back, bend the good leg and push that foot into the mattress in order to roll onto the 'bad' side.

Simple exercises, preferably after heat:

a) Lie on your back, bend first one knee up on to your chest and then put it down. Repeat with the other leg and alternate several times.

b) When standing, put your hands in the hollow of your back and arch backwards.

c) Relax whenever you can.

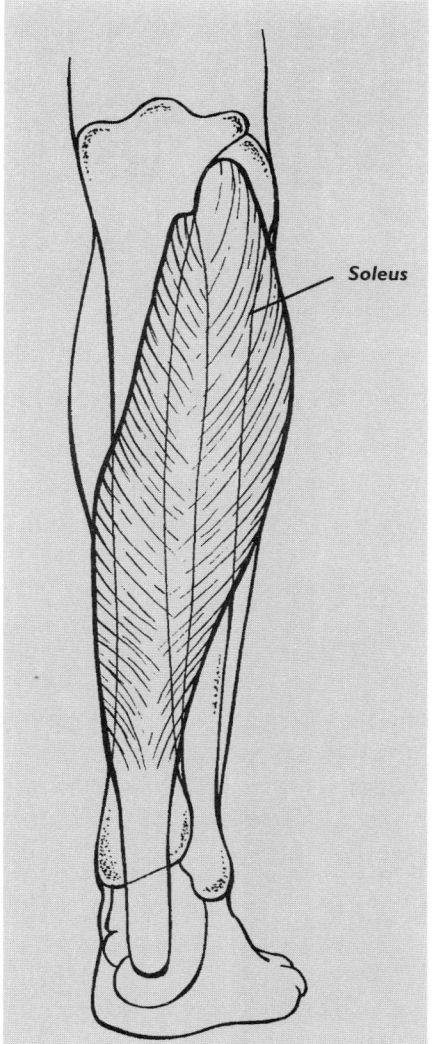

Figure Q: *Muscle of the calf*

The muscle of the calf – Soleus
(Figure Q)

Main Action: The muscle points the foot down when the knee is bent.

To minimise pain: If it is painful when you are sitting, get up and walk around.

Simple exercise, preferably after heat:

Work your foot up and down and round and round.

Chapter 16
EMERGENCY! I'M STUCK!

EMERGENCY!
I'm at the boot of the car.
I'm stuck! What do I do?

You are bending over the boot of the car, (see figure R (i)). Suddenly you are in excruciating pain. You cannot move, (see figure R (ii)). So:-

1) Don't panic.
   In this Body Language complaint, the cause most probably is the muscle having gone into acute spasm.

2) If you can, put a hand on the car and take the weight of your body through your hand, (see figure R (iii)).

3) *Stand still and breathe gently, rhythmically*, using the diaphragm. *Don't hold your breath.* Just wait until the acute muscle spasm wanes, as wane it will, (figure R (iii)).

4) When you feel able, bend the knees, (see figure R (iii)). This will bring the spine into a more vertical position.

5) Straighten the knees, (figure R (iv and v)).

Breathe in, breathe out, breathe in, breathe out, gently and rhythmically, all the time!

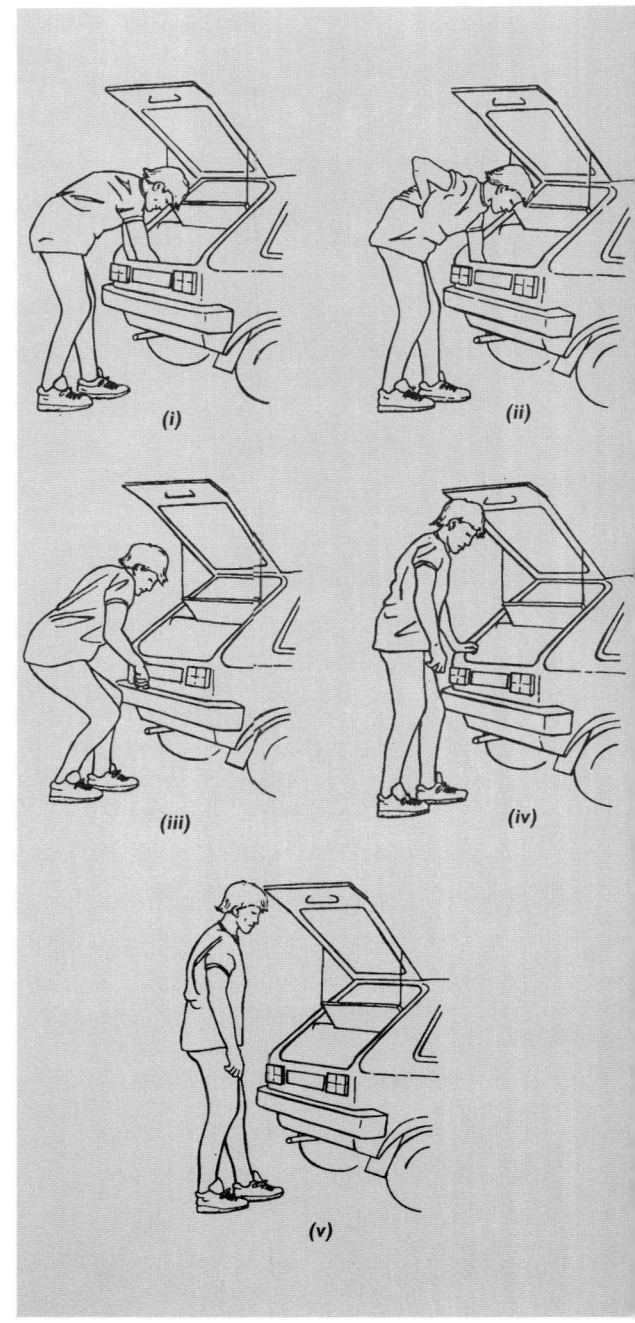

Figures R (i, ii, iii, iv and v): *Emergency at the car boot. What to do*

EMERGENCY!
Picking up a holdall or parcel from the floor.
I'm stuck! What do I do?

You are bending down to pick up a holdall, or a parcel, from the floor. Suddenly, you are in excruciating pain. You cannot move, (see S(i) and S(ii)). So:

1) Don't panic.
   In this Body Language complaint, the cause most probably is the muscle having gone into acute spasm.

2) If there is no handy chair or ledge to lean on, put your hands on the front of your thighs, and take the weight through them, (see figure S(iii)).

3) *Stand still. Breathe gently and rhythmically* with the diaphragm. *Don't hold your breath*. Just wait until the acute muscle spasm wanes, as wane it will.

4) Bend the knees, (figure S (iv)).

5) Walk the hands up the thighs, (figure S (v)).

6) Straighten the knees, (figure S (vi)).

Breathe in, breathe out, breathe in, breathe out, gently and rhythmically, all the time!

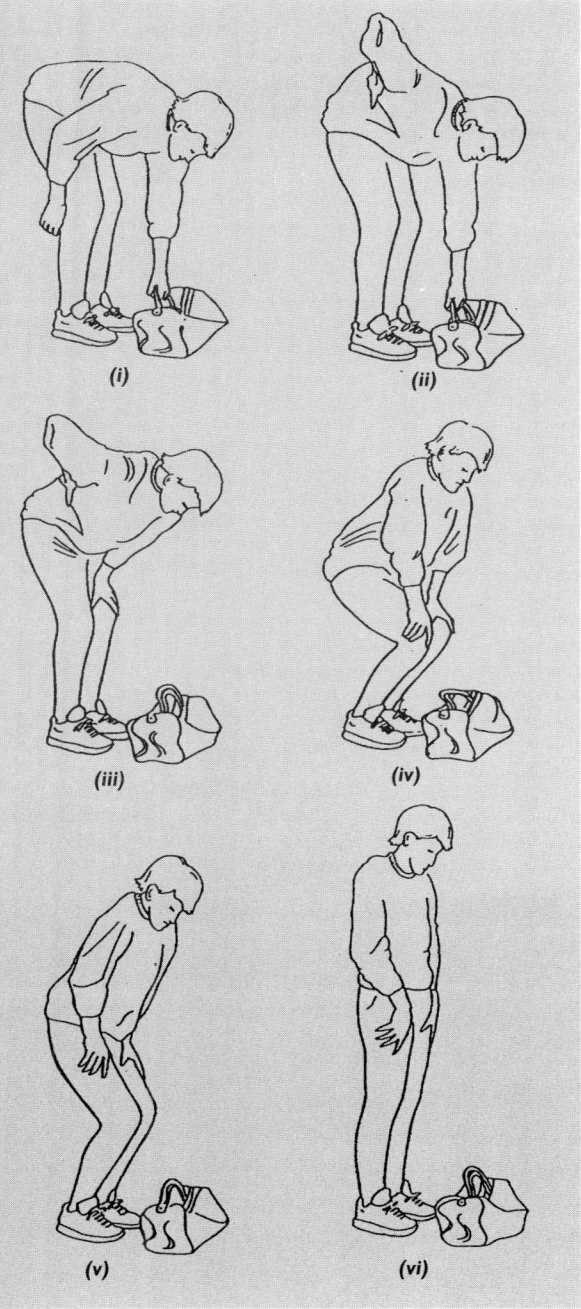

Figures S (i, ii, iii, iv, v and vi): Emergency when picking up a holdall or parcel

PART 2
OTHER PAINFUL PARTS

Chapter 17
Introduction

The first part of this book is about necks and backs. It shows how muscles in prolonged tension become painful. The muscles tense because of Body Language. Body Language is a reflex caused by our emotions. Our emotions are provoked by stress, and therefore stress causes muscle pain.

This same principle applies to other parts of the body. Other parts of the body also suffer pain from prolonged muscle tension, due to Body Language, resulting from our emotions, which are a reaction to stress.

This next section takes different parts of the body in turn, which suffer pain from prolonged muscle tension.

It is easier to divide it into parts of the body, than by the name of the painful condition, as there are often many names given for the one condition.

Each chapter will give the part of the body, then the common names, and then describe the condition. It will give details and diagrams of the muscles involved and their treatment; the Body Language and the stress that induces it. Lastly, it will give some examples of the causes of the condition with which patients suffer.

However, remember that to get the full understanding of any of these conditions, it is necessary to read, first of all, chapters 1 to 12. Then, read the particular chapter that interests you.

Chapter 18
Tennis Elbow and Golfer's Elbow

You should read chapters 1 to 12 first, and then continue here.

Tennis Elbow and Golfer's Elbow can be an injury to the elbow through playing either of these sports.

But it can also occur when there is no injury, no disease and in people who have never played either tennis or golf!

In the forearm there are 20 muscles doing things. We only want to find those which are causing trouble.

Of the 20 muscles, we are concerned with 10 of them, and these are the ones that go from your wrist and hand to either side of your elbow. Remember that your arm can twist (or rotate) in every direction and it has muscles going in every direction to allow you to do this.

There are those that go from the outside of the elbow down to the wrist and hand, and there are those that go from the inside of the elbow down to the wrist and hand ie. from the points of the elbow that we usually call the 'funny bone'. One of the elbow bones is called the humerus. Yes, that's why we call it the 'funny bone'!

What is it?
When we develop this condition, there is pain in the muscles of the forearm and sometimes swelling on the humerus. It can be painful when the arm is at rest. The pain can be increased when we grip hard and sometimes when we pick up something light, like a cup of tea.

a) Pain in the muscles.
The muscles which enable these actions to be performed are those in the forearm from the elbow to the wrist. These muscles tense even when not in use. Sometimes they feel hard. Sometimes only part of a muscle tenses, it looks normal and feels fairly soft. However, if the muscles tense wholly or partially, and *remain tense*, they become painful.

b) Swelling on the humerus.
This is called epicondylitis.
The muscles are attached to the humerus; the enlarged knobs on the humerus are called the epicondyles. The epicondyle swells. Why does the epicondyle become swollen?

Every bone, including the epicondyle, is covered in a sheath which is called the periosteum. The muscles actually adhere to this periosteum. When they tense, they pull on the periosteum. There are so many muscles attached to such a small area of the periosteum over the epicondyle that, when they are tense for a long time, the pull on the periosteum is so strong that it becomes damaged, inflamed and swollen.

This is the pain of Tennis or Golfer's Elbow.

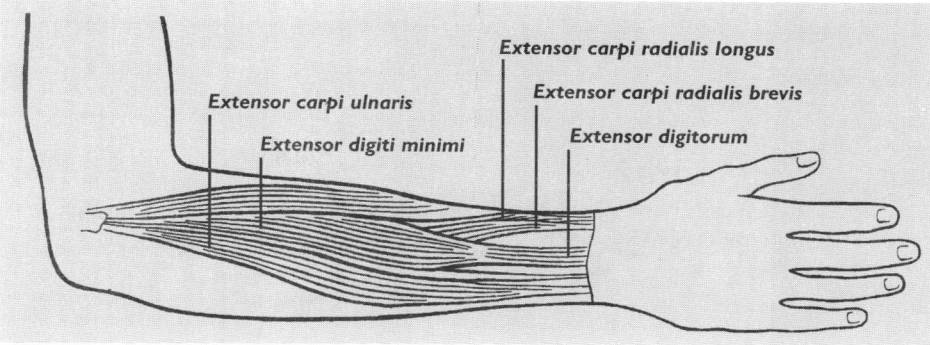

Figure T(i): Muscles of the forearm – the common extensors

Muscles involved in Tennis Elbow – the Common Extensors

The muscles involved are those which go from the outside of the elbow, down to the hand. There are 5 of them, all with long names. Fortunately, they are usually grouped together and simply referred to as the Common Extensors. See figure T(i).

Muscles in Golfer's Elbow – the Common Flexors

The muscles involved are those that go from the inside of the elbow down to the hand. There are 5 of them, also with long names, but are usually referred to as the Common Flexors. See figure T(ii).

Treatment of Tennis Elbow and Golfer's Elbow

Treatment must be to:

a) the tense muscles and

b) the inflamed periosteum.

a) Treatment of the muscles is aimed at their relaxation.
Heat, massage and relaxation, by the patient, helps. The treatment must be to the whole of the muscles, and not just the bit by the elbow.

The *patient* can help release the tension by making their own passive movements . They should 'flick' the wrist. To do this , the arm is held out at the side, with the elbow at a right angle, and the forearm suspended downwards.(See figure T(iii)).

Figure T(ii): Muscles of the forearm – the common flexors

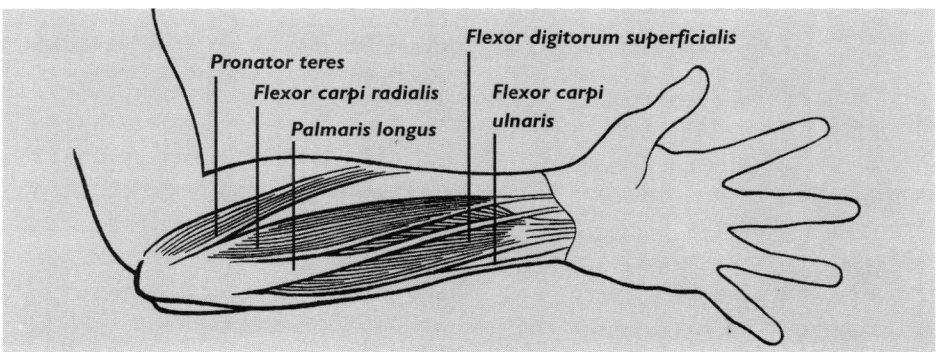

The arm is shaken so that the wrist flops backwards and forwards. It must be a floppy movement.

Between treatments check that you, the patient, are not inadvertently, clenching your fists; or holding things too tightly. For example, people often hold the car steering wheel far too tightly.

The patient frequently does not realise that the muscles of the forearm are tense.

The *physiotherapist* can help release the tension by passive movements to the muscles in the arms and legs. The movement of the legs in this instance, is only to enable the patient to learn the art of relaxation. It teaches the patient the sensation of relaxation. The passive movements can then be directed solely to the forearm.

b) Treatment of the Periosteum is aimed at reducing the swelling.

This is done by applying ice to the swelling. The simplest way is to use a small bag of frozen peas. First apply a thin paper tissue to the skin. Then apply the frozen peas. Wrap the elbow up in a towel, making sure that the peas are moulded to the elbow. Keep them there for fifteen minutes and do this three or four times a day.

Referred Pain

Pain itself, can be a source of stress. The muscles surrounding the painful condition may go into tension to protect the painful part. They themselves may become so tense that they are painful. The pain in this second group of tense and painful

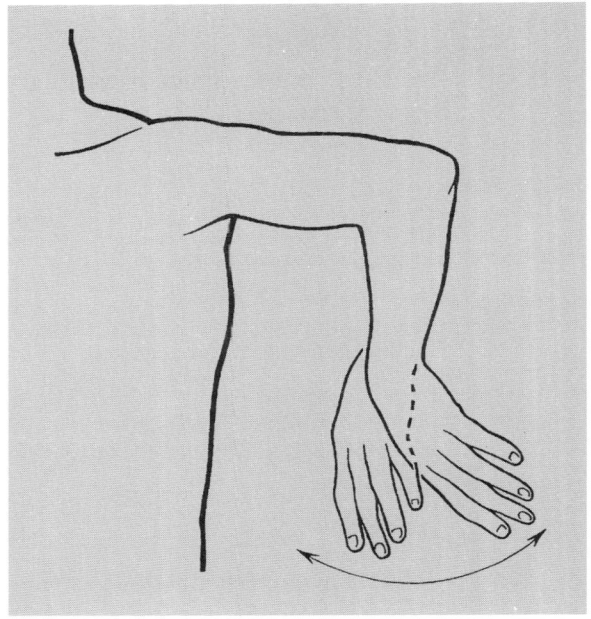

Figure T(iii): Flicking of the wrist

muscles is called referred pain. The muscles involved in referred pain are various. For instance they may involve Brachialis or Deltoid. They can be detected by a chartered physiotherapist. Treatment to them is aimed at promoting their relaxation.

At the beginning of this chapter, it was stated that this condition occurred in people who never played tennis or golf! But if that is so, what is the cause?

The Cause of Tennis Elbow and Golfer's Elbow
Why should the muscles involved in Tennis Elbow and Golfer's Elbow, tense?

Well here once again, we are talking about Body Language. Body Language and stress. "Stress?", I hear you say! "Stress causing tennis elbow?".

Human beings are very practical and to be practical, we use our hands. The hands can do such diverse things as wield a pickaxe, or play a piano. We regard them as very clever pieces of engineering, totally under our control.

However, the hands do, subconsciously, clench when we are stressed. We see people, whom we know to be tense, with their fists clenched. It is quite a common sight. This kind of fist clenching is Body Language; Body Language affecting the muscles according to how we feel. The clenching is brought about by the same muscles which are affected in Tennis and Golfer's Elbow.

So much for the muscles. But what kind of emotion makes us clench our fists?

The emotion results from the kind of stress caused where our position is threatened, and we still try to keep what we've got. Verbally, we express ourselves by the phrases, "Hold tight", or "Hang on there".

Look at the picture of the woman sitting on the chair. (Figure T(iv))

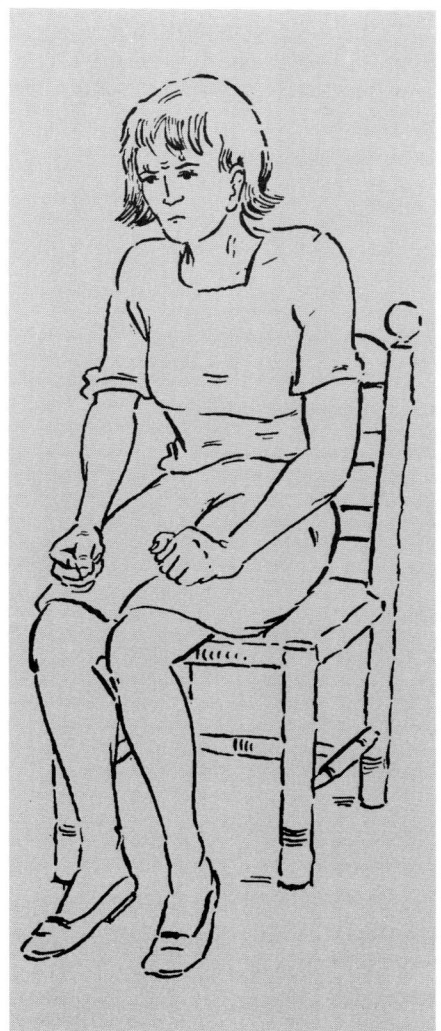

Figure T(iv)

What does her Body Language tell us? It tells us that she is tense. How do we know? Because her fists are clenched. We often see people do this, and accept it as an outward sign of inner tension.

"Hold tight" or "Hang on there", are phrases that we use to encourage people to keep going in times of difficulty.

Well, we may be stressed; we may be "hanging on". But we certainly don't look like that woman in the picture! We look normal, calm and in control of ourselves. Great.

However, if we are stressed and "hanging on", even though we bottle up our emotions and carry on as normal, the muscles which clench the fists, even though not visible to the eye, are still tense. This is subconscious, a reflex action and outside our control. They may not tense enough to bring about visible clenching, but even partially tensed muscles, if they *remain tense*, will become painful.

To summarise, treatment of Tennis Elbow and Golfer's Elbow must be directed at both the elbow and the forearm. The cause of this complaint is the stress inducing Body Language. It follows, therefore, that it is only when the cause itself has been finally resolved or the attitude to the stress is changed so that it is no longer a stress, or the stress has been completely forgotten that a final cure will be effected.

Examples
The examples are suitably disguised.

1) The man who inherited a family furnishing business was , because of the economic climate, finding that his business was going down. He developed 'Tennis Elbow', desperately 'clinging on' to his business.

2) The woman, who resigned her full time job , and set up on her own as a self employed management consultant, developed pain in the elbow. The pain was on both sides of the elbow and so was diagnosed as Tennis and Golfer's Elbow. Every week she counted her meagre earnings, and multiplied the figure by 52 to see how much she would earn in a year. She was worried sick that she would not bring in enough money to earn her living; but she 'clung on' to her new business hoping that clients would come to her, so that her business would thrive and she would become a success.

Neither of these two people played tennis or golf. Sometimes they would visibly clench their fists, although they themselves were unaware of this. Sometimes the fists would not be clenched. However, the muscles causing the clenching action would still partially tense – not enough to bring about visible clenching, but for long enough to become painful.

Chapter 19
Pain in the Shoulder
sometimes called
Frozen Shoulder

You should read chapters 1 to 12 first, then continue here.

What is it?
Frozen shoulder is the painful condition in the shoulder where there has been no injury, and there is no disease.

Frozen shoulder is an umbrella term used to describe three variations of this painful condition in the shoulder:

a) where the shoulder is painful, but the joint is not stiff,

b) where the shoulder is painful and the joint is stiff,

c) where there is no pain in the shoulder, but the joint is stiff.

a) Where the shoulder is painful, but the joint is not stiff.
When you have a frozen shoulder, it hurts to lift things, it hurts to put on your coat, it hurts to reach for your seat belt, it hurts, sometimes, to do the simplest things, such as reaching out of your car window to take the car parking ticket from the machine. It also hurts when you are not moving at all! In this condition, the pain is in the muscles. The muscles become tense, remain tense, and so become painful.

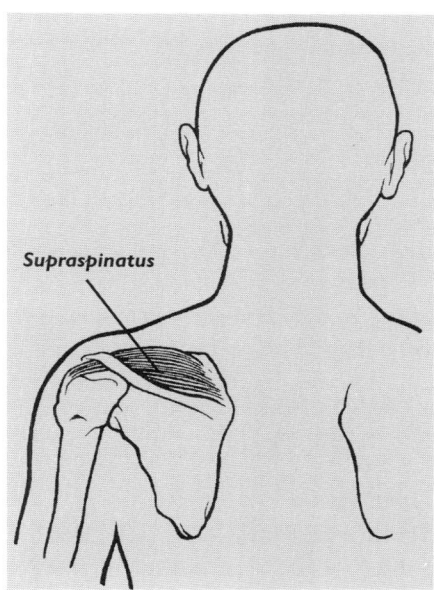

Figure U(i): Muscle of the shoulder

Muscles involved in Frozen Shoulder
There are two main muscles involved. One lies across the top of the shoulder, and is called Supraspinatus. (See figure U(i)).

The other lies like a cloak round the shoulder and is called Deltoid.
(See figure U(ii) and U(iii)).

Treatment
Treatment of these muscles is aimed at making them relax. Heat and massage and relaxation by the patient, and passive movements by the physiotherapist are both aimed at inducing relaxation. (See chapter 10.)

If the pain is agonising, rest the arm in a sling for a couple of days.

Simple exercise, preferably after heat. Whilst doing any of the following exercises, never hold your breath. Breathe slowly, rhythmically, not too deeply and breathe with the diaphragm.

Shrugging of the shoulders helps to loosen the area generally. Moving the arms is, at first, painful, I'm afraid. However, if you can persevere, it does help ease the tension and so ease the pain.

With a frozen shoulder it is helpful for the patient to swing the arm forwards and backwards half a dozen times. Progress this to swinging it round and round, rhythmically, like a windmill.

Useful Tips
If working at a desk, make sure that it is the right height. If it is too high, it will make the pain worse.

Do not carry a shoulder bag on the painful side. Do not lift weights.

b) Where the shoulder is painful and the joint is stiff.

The pain in the shoulder may be so acute that it is impossible to move, however willing the patient is to try. This means that the shoulder joint has not moved. If a joint is kept immobile, then simply through non use, it will become stiff.

There are now two problems – pain in the muscles *and* a stiff joint. Treatment then has to have two approaches:

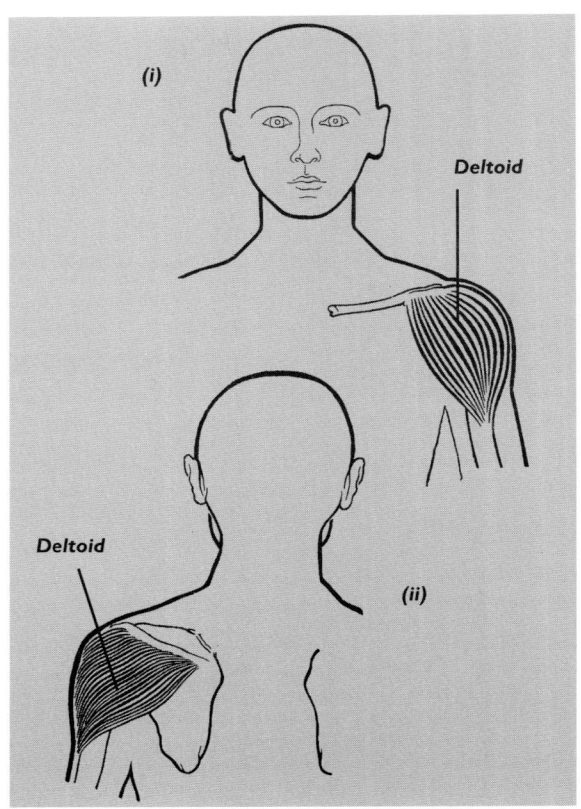

Figure U(ii and iii): *Muscle of the shoulder*

i) treatment to the muscle, as already described, and

ii) treatment to the joint.

The shoulder must be warm and has to be encouraged to move. This is done, using the good arm. Either sit down, or lie down on a bed. Hold the hands together. Raise the arms up above the head, the good arm taking the weight. When you have gone as far as you can, bring the arms down. Repeat this movement several times, taking the arms up a bit higher each time. If the joint is too stiff for the exercise, you should consult a chartered physiotherapist.

Whilst doing any of the exercises, never hold your breath. Breathe slowly, rhythmically, not too deeply, and breathe with the diaphragm.

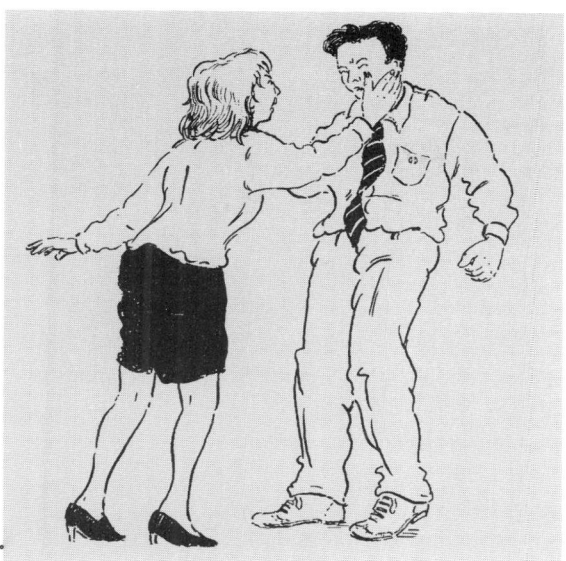

Figure U(iv)

c) Where there is no pain in the shoulder, but the joint is stiff.
On its own, this is not a muscle tension problem and you should consult your doctor.

However, where the pain from tense muscles is so acute that you cannot move your shoulder, the joint will become stiff through non use.

If the muscle pain is then cured, you may be left with a stiff joint.

The exercises in the previous paragraph, when describing treatment of painful and stiff joints, should be carried out. If the joint is too stiff for the exercises, you should consult a chartered physiotherapist.

Referred Pain
There may be additional muscles which are painful. They are muscles which tense, in order to protect the painful part, but in so doing, may become so tense that they, themselves, become painful. The pain in this second group of tense and painful muscles is called referred pain. The muscles involved, in referred pain, are various. They might be Rectus Capitis Major and Minor, Levator Scapulae, Extensors of the wrist, Brachialis, Pronator Teres or Pectoralis Major. They can be detected by a chartered physiotherapist. In all cases, treatment to them is aimed at promoting their relaxation.

The Cause
Why should these muscles at the shoulder, tense?
The muscles tense through Body Language. Body Language is a reaction to our emotions.

What kind of emotion could affect the shoulder? Look at the picture, figure U(iv).

There will be plenty of emotion in a girl who slaps a man's face! Whatever the reason! There will be emotion in a man who hits another man (see figure U(v)).

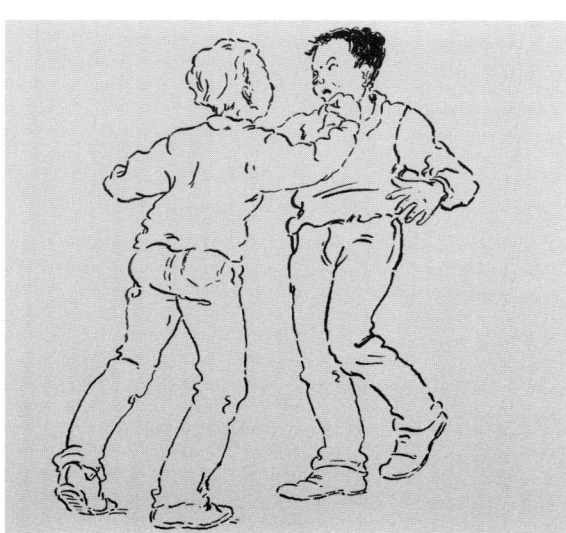

Figure U(v)

However, most of us don't go round hitting people. It's not the best way to make friends! But we do hear people say, with great feeling, "Ooh, I could hit him!", or " I could slap his face". This is a natural emotion.

Nevertheless, it is not a good idea to hit someone. It may make the situation worse. It may even land us in trouble with the law!

So we restrain our actions, and we bottle up our emotions.

However, if this emotion is strong and continues for some time, especially where we are not able to do much about it, the muscles which would drive forward the action are the shoulder muscles and these would tense involuntarily. It is a reflex action and outside our control. If the muscles *remain tense*, they become painful.

We have talked about treatment of the muscles which eases the pain and may get rid of it completely for a time. However, there will only be a permanent removal of the pain if:

a)   the stress ceases, or

b)   the person changes their attitude to it, so that it is no longer a stress to them, or

c)   they forget the stress completely.

Examples
What kind of incident produces this? Well there are an infinite number. What annoys one person does not necessarily annoy another. However, here are two examples – both suitably disguised.

1) The man who worked in a large engineering firm had, by the nature of his job, to do a certain amount of entertaining. He submitted one set of expense claims, but they were reduced by the accounts department. After that, all his expense claims were subject to minute scrutiny by the accounts department. The engineer felt he was being unfairly criticised and was always on the defence about his expenses. After all, he was away from home a lot on business; he worked long hours and travelled a lot. Not like the people in the office questioning his expenses! He developed a frozen shoulder, because he was frustrated by bureaucracy and he wanted to hit back.

2) An eighteen year old girl lived at home with her widowed mother and younger sister. The mother always discussed the running of the house with, and took notice of, the younger girl's opinion. The eighteen year old girl, whose opinions were always dismissed, felt hurt and on the defence because she did not know why. She was frustrated; she loved her mum; she couldn't hurt her or even shout at her. She developed pain in the shoulder muscles, as she wanted to hit back.

Chapter 20
Pain round the side of the Chest Wall
sometimes called
Fibrositis or Fibromyalgia

You should read chapters 1 to 12 first, and then continue here.

What is it?

Again, this is not pain resulting from any disease, nor from any injury. When people get pain round the side of the chest wall, they immediately think that there is something wrong with their heart or lungs. This obviously has to be checked out with the doctor, as with all unknown pain.

If the doctor says that there is nothing wrong with the heart and lungs and that the pain is in the muscle, we are looking at a not very well known muscle which lies round the side of the chest, underneath the arm. This can become tense, and if it *remains tense*, it becomes painful.

Muscle involved

The muscle involved is the Serratus Anterior. (See figures V(i) and V(ii)).

On the back of the ribs is the scapula, or shoulder blade. This bone is shaped like a flat triangular plate. The Serratus anterior is attached to the underneath side of the scapula, reaches round the side of the chest wall, and attaches to the ribs at the front. The scapula works in close connection with the arm. This means that when the arm is pushing forward, the scapula is also moving and it is the Serratus anterior muscle which is moving the scapula. You cannot prod this muscle with your finger, where it lies underneath the bony scapula but you can prod it, underneath the arm, as it comes round the side of the chest to the front.

Treatment

By the patient. The aim of treatment is to ease the tension in the muscle. Heat and massage and relaxation techniques by the patient are helpful. See chap10.

By the therapist. Passive movements of the arm and scapula by the therapist help to reduce the tension, and at the

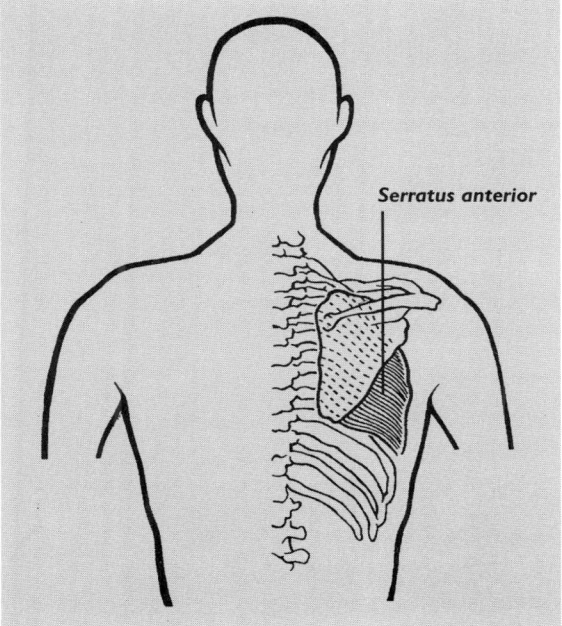

Figure V(i): *muscle round the chest wall*

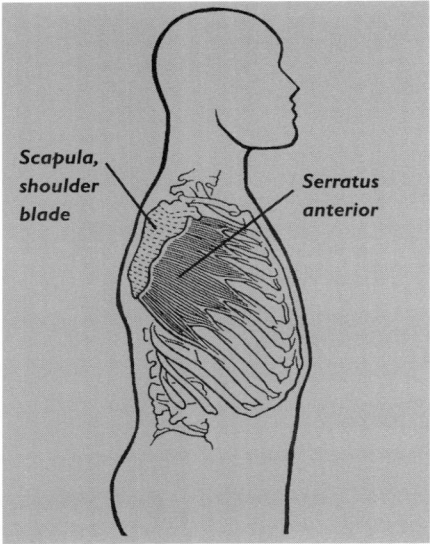

Figure V(ii): Muscle round the chest wall

same time teach the patient what is required by relaxation. See chapter 10.

Simple exercise, preferably after heat.
The scapula and the arm are closely connected. So when the arm moves, the scapula moves too, involving the Serratus Anterior muscle.

1) When lying or sitting, brace the shoulder blades back, and then relax. Repeat this half a dozen times. Then let your arms hang by your side, and breathe gently with the diaphragm. Repeat the exercise if necessary.

2) Swing the arms forwards and backwards, slowly swinging the arms higher and higher half a dozen times. Then relax.

Whilst doing either of the exercises never hold your breath. Breathe slowly, rhythmically, not too deeply and breathe with the diaphragm.

Useful Tip
Don't carry weights while the pain is severe.

Referred Pain
Pain itself can be a source of stress. The muscles surrounding the painful condition may go into tension to protect the painful part. They themselves may become so tense that they are painful. The pain in this second group of tense and painful muscles is called referred pain and might involve Supraspinatus, Deltoid, Quadratus lumborum or Iliocostalis. The muscles involved in referred pain can be detected by a chartered physiotherapist. In any case, treatment to them is aimed at promoting their relaxation.

The Cause
Why does the muscle round the chest wall, tense?
The muscle, Serratus anterior, tenses to the point of pain due to Body Language.

"Body Language round the chest wall?", I can hear you ask. " I thought that Body Language showed different postures according to our emotions, and there's none of that round the chest wall".

But there is posture from emotion, when using our arms.

Look at the picture of the man pushing away the other man. See figure V(iii).

There's emotion there! – his Body Language is telling the other man to move away.

Sometimes, when we want someone to move away from us, we say to them, "push off", (or another less polite phrase!).

PAIN ROUND THE SIDE OF THE CHEST WALL

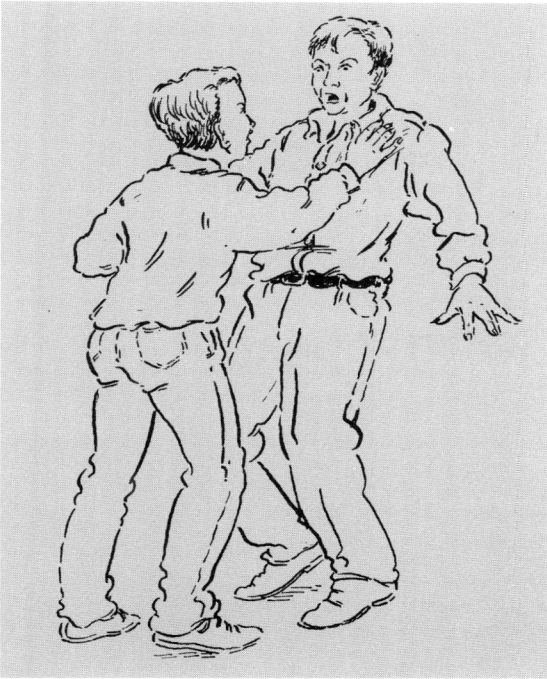

Figure V(iii)

"I need space"; "I need room"; "Give me air"; "Get out of my hair"; "Go and take a running jump," are all phrases we use in order to tell someone to move away from us.

However, pushing them, or even telling them to push off, is not always the correct social thing to do. So we don't do it, but if it is what we want, the muscle which does the pushing ie. Serratus anterior, will still tense. If it *remains tense*, it will become painful. This tension is a reflex, is totally subconscious and is outside our control.

We have talked about treatment of the muscles, which eases the pain, and may get rid of it completely for a time. However, there will only be a permanent removal of the pain if:

a) the stress ceases, or

b) the person changes their attitude to it, so that it is no longer a stress to them, or

c) they forget it completely.

Examples

The examples are suitably disguised.

1) A young married woman had a widowed father. She and her husband were fond of him. However, he was always round at their house and they never had a weekend on their own. They wanted time on their own; they wanted their own space. They wished he would not come so often. His daughter wanted to push him away and developed pain round the chest wall, in the Serratus anterior muscle.

2) A wife, reluctantly, had her unfriendly mother-in-law to stay for the weekend. During the weekend, the mother-in-law made several hurtful remarks about her, and the way she ran her house. The wife, who was annoyed, longed to push her mother-in-law back home, out of the way. She could not do that as she had invited her, and so developed pain round the chest wall.

Chapter 21
Pain in the Front of the Ribs
sometimes called
Intercostal Myalgia or Neuralgia or Pleurodynia

You should read chapters 1 to 12 first, and then continue here.

What is it?
Intercostal myalgia is pain that has nothing to do with any injury, nor with any disease in the chest or abdomen. It is a pain with a cramp like feeling and it occurs at the front of the ribs, just to the side of the breast bone or sternum. At the front of the chest, behind the ribs and just to the side of the sternum, lies a small muscle which stretches from behind the sternum to the adjoining ribs, (figure W(i)). Because of its position it is not possible to prod it with your finger. Sometimes this muscle tenses, *remains tense*, and so it becomes painful.

Muscle involved
The muscle is the Transversus Thoracis (see figure W(i)).

The job of this muscle is to draw the ribs down and inwards, to force air out of our lungs, as we do when we are crying. This action helps to produce the deep sobs of crying.

Treatment
Apply local heat, such as a hot water bottle, on the ribs. Massage is virtually impossible, as the muscle lies underneath the ribs. Relieving the tension in the muscle is helped by a

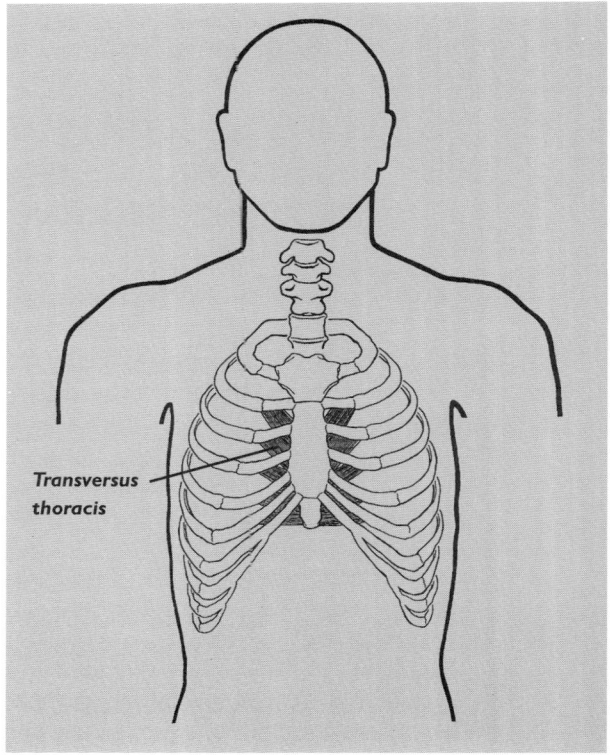

Figure W(i): *Muscle at the front of the ribs*

breathing exercise. The breathing is aimed at expanding the lower ribs, so elongating the tense Transversus thoracis muscle.

Breathing exercise
Breathe in, so that the abdomen comes forward, and the rib cage expands to the side, as far as possible. This helps

PAIN IN THE FRONT OF THE RIBS

to release the tension in the Transversus thoracis muscle. Then relax and breathe out. Repeat this half a dozen times, then have a rest. If the pain is still there, repeat the breathing once more. If it remains, rest, and then do it again say, one hour later.

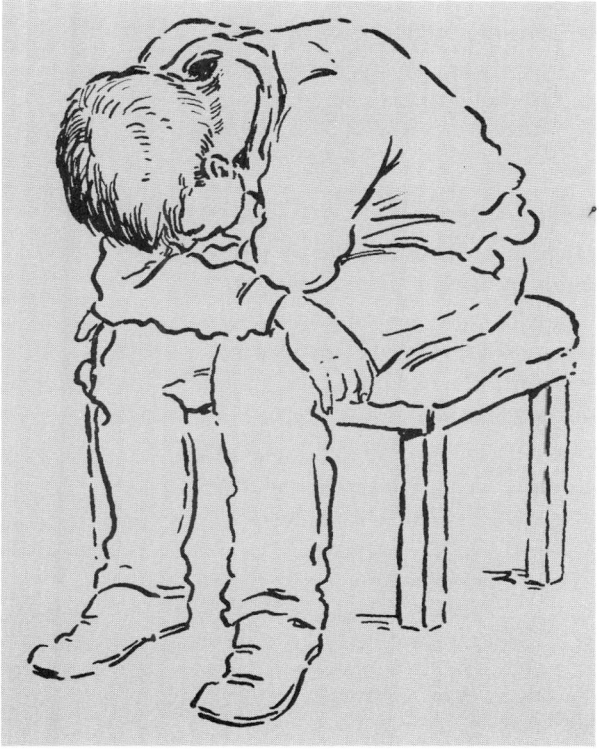

Figure W(ii)

After you have done this exercise, don't hold your breath. Breathe slowly, rhythmically, and not too deeply.

The Cause
Why do we get this pain at the front of the ribs, called intercostal myalgia?
The answer lies in Body Language. "Body Language in our ribs?" Hard to imagine!

Perhaps it would be easier to understand if you looked at the picture of the boy sitting on the stool, figure W(ii).

What does it indicate? – total dejection. His body is slumped down towards his thighs.

He is crying and you can see from his Body Language that he is feeling utterly wretched, and forlorn, his sobs coming in short strangled bursts. The sobs are brought about by the air being forced out of the lungs.

The muscle which pulls the ribs down to expel the air, lies at the front of the chest and behind the lower ribs and, as stated previously, is the Transversus thoracis. (See figure W(i)).

Fortunately this extreme and acute depression is quite rare with most people. However, life is not always happy. There are occasions when we do feel sad – not sad enough to force us to collapse on a chair and cry – but sad, nevertheless.

On these occasions, we continue with our daily tasks. The action of crying is suppressed, but the Transversus thoracis muscle which brings about the crying, still tenses. It tenses as a reflex; it tenses outside our control. If it *remains tense*, it gets to the point of pain which is called intercostal myalgia.

We have talked about treatment of the muscle, which eases the pain, and may get rid of it completely for a time. However, there will only be a permanent removal of the pain, if:

a) the stress ceases, or

b) the person changes their attitude to it, so that it is no longer a stress to them, or

c) they forget it completely.

Examples

What circumstances can produce this? Here are two examples – both suitably disguised. The one thing common to both, is their feeling of sadness.

1) A widower had pain in the chest wall on the first anniversary of his much loved wife's death. On this day the memories of her death were particularly poignant. He went to work as usual but kept thinking of her and so felt very sad. He developed intercostal myalgia.

2) A girl was engaged to be married to a man of whom her mother strongly disapproved. She went to meet her mother in order to have a heart to heart talk, but was unable to convince her mother that he was the right man for her, and left the meeting feeling miserable and sad. On the way home, she developed acute pain in the ribs which is called intercostal myalgia.

Chapter 22
Pain in the Groin and Down the Front of the Thigh
sometimes called
Groin pain or Fibromyalgia or Anterior Knee Pain

You should read chapters 1 to 12 first, and then continue here.

What is it?
It is pain, an aching pain extending from the groin down to the knee. It may be in the groin only; it may be in the front of the thigh; it may be down the inside of the thigh or it may be down the outside of the thigh.

We are not talking about pain that is the result of any injury or any disease. We are discussing the pain that is in the muscles due to the muscles being tense. The pain may be felt when we are not moving at all. It may be felt when the muscles have to work in order to perform movements.

When tense and painful muscles are made to contract in order to make us move, they become even more painful. This is very noticeable in these leg muscles.

Movements, like walking, running, climbing stairs, coming down stairs, bending the knees into a crouch position, lifting the knee to put on a sock, crossing the legs when sitting, placing the feet together when standing up straight, or even just standing up straight, can be very painful. In fact these movements can be so excruciatingly painful that you cannot do them at all.

There are a number of muscles involved in this area. Which movement causes pain, depends on which muscle is involved.

Muscles Involved
The following muscles are involved, sometimes separately, sometimes with each other.

They are:

Psoas and Iliacus, see figure X(i)
Rectus Femoris, see figure X(ii)
Adductor muscles, see figure X(iv)
Tensor Fasciae Latae, see figure X(v)

Treatment
The aim of treatment is relaxation of the muscles. (See chapter 10.)

Treatment by the patient
The treatment includes heat and massage to the muscle. Massaging the muscles of the thighs is easier than massaging the muscles in your back – at least you can reach your thighs. Follow this by relaxing the muscles. Let the limbs feel heavy and floppy. Breathe with the diaphragm slowly, rhythmically and not too deeply. Think about the breathing. See chapter 10.

Psoas and Iliacus muscles (Xi)
With Psoas and Iliacus muscles, sit up, with your back well supported, and put three pillows under your knees. This is to take the strain and put the muscles in a slack position. The muscles lie deep in the groin, so the massage needs to be small circular movements with your fingers, into the groin, as deep as you can.

Simple exercise, preferably after heat.
1) Stand on your good leg, hold onto a firm piece of furniture, swing the affected leg backwards and forwards, half a dozen times, with slightly more emphasis on swinging backwards. Make it as much of a relaxed movement as you can. Breathe with your diaphragm while you are doing it.

2) Mark time on the spot, half a dozen times; don't lift the legs up high in the front – the feet should only just leave the ground. Start slowly, gradually mark time a little quicker.

Useful Tips
1) When in bed lie with the knees propped up, or resting over three pillows.

2) When sitting in a chair bend the knees up, or put them over the arm of the chair.

3) Don't try to run when the pain is acute.

4) Do walk slowly with short steps, swinging the legs in as relaxed a way as you can.

5) Go up stairs one at a time, with the good leg first.

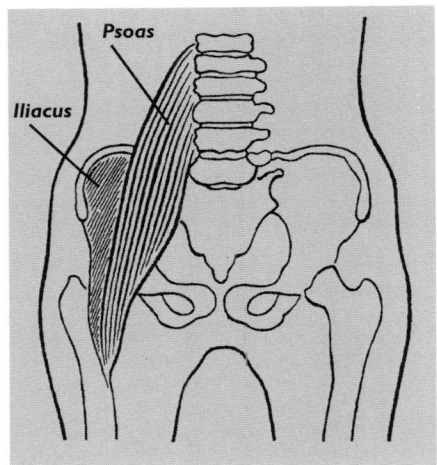
Figure X(i): Muscles of the groin

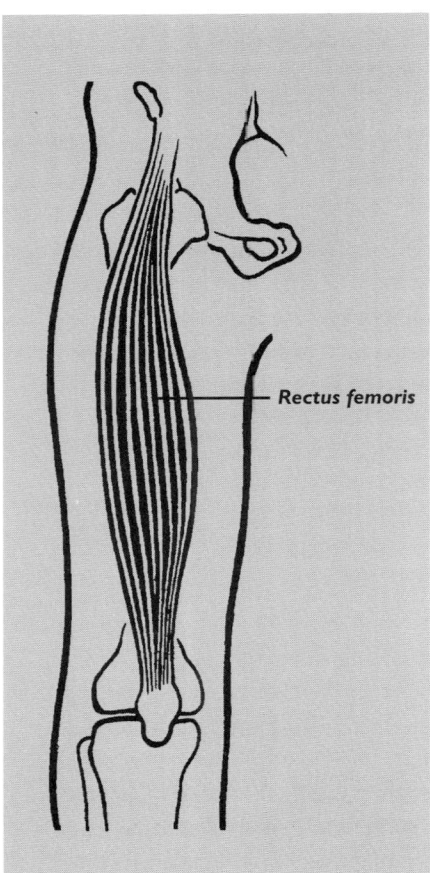
Figure X(ii): Muscles of the thigh

PAIN IN THE GROIN AND DOWN THE FRONT OF THE THIGH

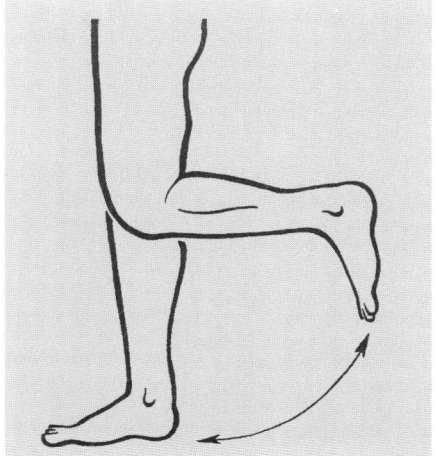

Figure X(iii): Bending the knee backwards

Rectus Femoris muscle (Xii)
Rectus femoris is a long muscle stretching from the front of the hip to just below the knee and it lies just under the skin. Circular kneading massage helps, as does long firm stroking of the muscle.

Simple exercise, preferably after heat.
1) Stand on your good leg, hold onto a firm piece of furniture, swing the affected leg backwards and forwards with slightly more emphasis on swinging backwards. Make it as much of a relaxed movement as you can. Breathe with your diaphragm while you are doing it.

2) Mark time on the spot; don't lift the legs up high in the front, the feet should only just leave the ground. Start slowly, gradually mark time a little quicker.

3) Stand and lift one foot backwards so that the knee bends. Repeat with alternate legs. See figure X(iii).

Useful Tips
1) When in bed lie with the knees and the calfs resting over three pillows.

2) When sitting on a chair, bend the knees up, or put them over the arm of the chair.

3) Don't try to run when the pain is bad.

4) Do walk slowly with short steps, swinging the legs in as relaxed a way as is possible.

5) Go up stairs one at a time, the good leg always goes first; go down one at a time, the bad leg always goes first.

Adductor muscles (X(iv))
The Adductor muscles lie just under the skin on the inside of the thigh, from the groin down to the knee, so it is easy to massage them. Circular movements and long firm strokes can be helpful.

Simple exercise, preferably after heat.
1) Stand on your good leg, hold onto a firm piece of furniture, swing the affected leg from the standing position, outwards and back, half a dozen times. Make it as much of a relaxed movement as you can. Breathe with the diaphragm whilst swinging.

2) Mark time on the spot, half a dozen times. Don't lift the legs up high in the front. The feet should only just leave the ground. Start slowly, gradually mark time a little quicker.

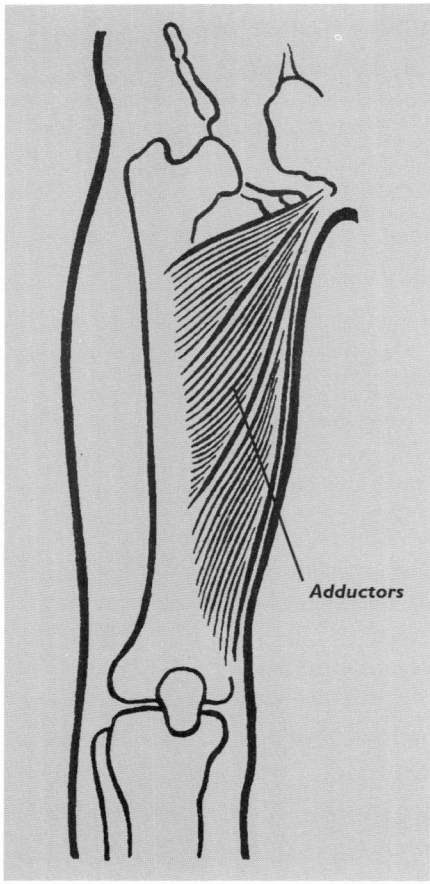

Figure X(iv): Muscles of the thigh

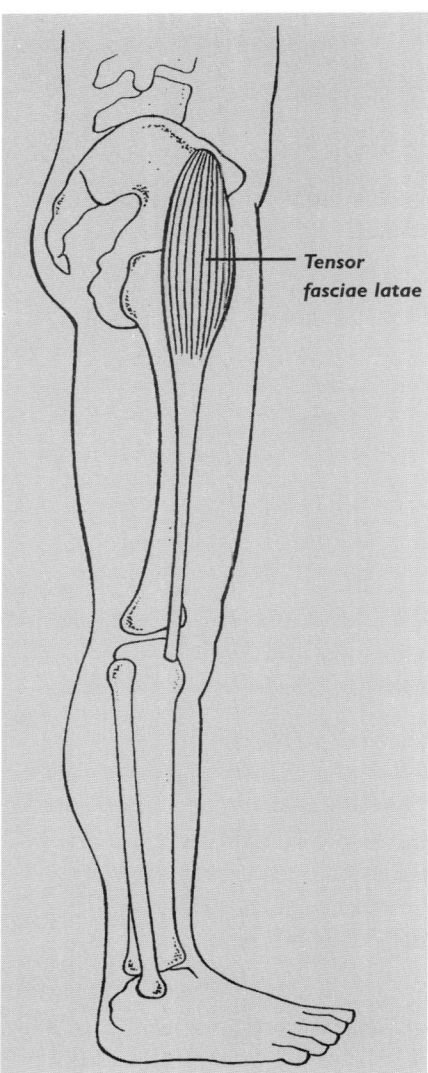

Figure X(v): Muscles of the thigh

Useful Tips

1) Don't try to run if the pain is bad.

2) Do walk slowly with short steps, swinging the legs in as relaxed a way as you can.

3) When standing, stand with your feet about four inches apart.

Tensor Fasciae Latae muscle (X(v))
Tensor fasciae latae muscle has been described under the section on Backache. However, it is included here as the pain in a Tensor Fasciae Latae muscle is often felt by the patient only at its lower end, that is, at the side of the knee. This is why it is occasionally described as Anterior Knee Pain. Massage of this muscle needs to be along its entire length, down the whole of the outside of the thigh and not just at the lower end. Circular movements

and long stroking movements may be helpful.

Simple exercise, preferably after heat.
Sit or lie with the leg outstretched. Rotate, or roll, the leg in and out fairly vigorously, half a dozen times. Finish with it rotated out. Then relax it as much as you can. Repeat as necessary.

Useful Tips
1) In bed when lying on your side, place two fat pillows between the knees.

2) Stand with your feet well apart when standing.

Whilst doing any of the exercises with any of these muscles, never hold your breath. Breathe slowly, rhythmically, not too deeply and breathe with the diaphragm.

Treatment by the physiotherapist
The aim of treatment to Psoas, Iliacus, Rectus femoris, Adductors and Tensor fasciae latae is to achieve relaxation of the muscle. This involves moving various parts of the body in a slow rhythmical and repetitive way, and then concentrating on the legs and their muscles. There should not be any forced or jerking movements. At the same time, the patient lets the legs and even the arms and head, go totally limp. See chapter 10.

Referred pain
There may also be additional muscles that are painful. They are muscles which tense in order to protect the painful part. They may become so tense that they are painful. The pain in this second group of tense and painful muscles is called referred pain. The muscles involved in referred pain vary. They might be Extensor digitorum longus, Peroneus longus and brevis, Soleus, Psoas, Iliacus, Pectineus, or Adductor brevis and they can be detected by a chartered physiotherapist. Treatment to them is aimed at promoting their relaxation.

So we have muscles in the groin and the thigh which may become tense, and through *prolonged tension*, become painful. But if this can come about without disease and without injury, why does it occur?

The Cause
Why do the muscles tense in the groin and at the front of the thigh?
They tense, until they become painful, because of Body Language. Body Language is the way that we subconsciously hold our body, as a response to our emotions. It may be thought that emotion is shown only on our faces or expressed with our hands. However, other parts of the body are equally responsive to our emotions.

Look at the picture of the little boy kicking the adult, (figure X(vi)).

He is obviously cross with the adult. He clearly does not like the woman, or perhaps does not like what she stands for. So he kicks her. A little child who does not agree with his friend might kick him. It is a form of aggressive behaviour that is often seen in a playground.

Kicking someone is anti-social. It is not acceptable in an adult. Adults don't kick people – usually! However, 'kicking against authority', is a phrase which we often hear; a phrase which does describe our emotions. But we learn to control our emotions, or at least the outer manifestations of them. Nevertheless, if we are feeling aggressive, we will still have the urge to give someone a 'good kick in the pants'. Even if we do not show our emotions, the muscles which perform the kick, that is those in the groin and the thigh, will still tense. They tense as a reflex reaction, which is outside our control. With the feeling of aggression, comes the natural muscle tension. If the aggressive emotion in us persists, the muscles will remain tense. If the muscles *remain tense*, they will become painful.

We have talked about the treatment of the muscles, which eases the pain, and may get rid of it completely for a time. However, there will only be a permanent removal of the pain if:

a) the stress ceases or,

b) the person changes their attitude to it, so that it is no longer a stress to them or,

c) they forget it completely.

Examples
The examples are suitably disguised.

1) An author wrote a novel, submitted it to a publisher who neither refused nor accepted it for publication. The publisher could not decide. The author, whilst waiting for a decision, developed pain in the front of the groin and thigh, 'kicking' the publisher to

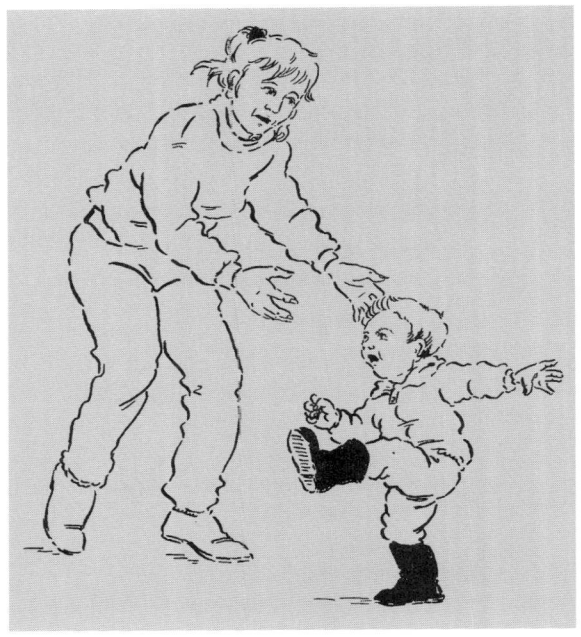

Figure X(vi)

decide in his favour. "Go on, publish it" he was silently urging.

2) A very efficient office worker was told by her superior, that she deserved promotion and he would put in a good word with the proprietor of the firm on her behalf. However the proprietor would not make up his mind. He kept procrastinating about her promotion. She developed pain down the front of her thighs. "I wish he would make up his mind", she said "I could kick him!".

Chapter 23
Massage

Massage is a useful form of treatment for muscle pain and it can be done by the patient themselves or by a willing relative or friend.

Many patients try to get their husbands or wives to do the massage for them, but find that the new 'masseur' is either scared to death of hurting them and hardly dare touch them, or is so enthusiastic, that the patient is nearly pushed through the bed! The 'masseur' may dig the fingers in so deeply that the pain is made even worse.

Perhaps the need for massage needs to be explained.

Why do we massage the muscles?
We massage the muscles because we want to get rid of the pain, and this is one way of doing it. The pain is due to muscle tension , so we want to get rid of the tension and get the muscles relaxed. One way to get the muscles relaxed is to give *soothing* massage. It can be a pleasant sensation and so be an antidote to pain. Because it is a pleasant sensation, it can help to induce relaxation. Relaxation itself, is very important.

Massage also increases the circulation and so helps to get rid of the excess lactic acid which builds up in the muscle when it is tense.

PREPARATION FOR MASSAGE

Preparation of the patient
Before beginning the massage, *the patient has to be made comfortable*. You can massage someone while they are standing up, or while they are sitting on the edge of a stool, but this won't help them to relax because, if they did relax, they would fall down!

Get the patient sitting or lying down, get them comfortable; support their limbs with pillows; make sure that they are warm. They cannot relax if they are shivering.

For massage to the neck and shoulders, elbow and forearm
Sit the patient on a chair with a cushion behind the back. Put a cushion on their knees so that their arms can rest on the pillow.

For massage to the neck only
Another position for the patient with a neck problem is to lie on a bed on their back, with the head at the foot of the bed so that the neck can be reached. The masseur stands behind the patient.

For massage to the back
Lie the patient face downwards if they can get into this position. Place one or two pillows underneath the abdomen first, and then place one under the shins and feet.

If they cannot lie face down, lie them on their side, with a pillow under the head and another pillow between the knees.

For massage to the side of the chest
Lie the patient on their side with the painful side of the chest uppermost. Place a pillow under the head, one between the knees and one in front of the chest. The pillow in front of the chest is to support their upper arm.

Preparation of the masseur
The next stage is to *make the masseur comfortable*.

No masseur can massage for a long time, or even for five minutes, if they are having to stoop or reach beyond their natural stance. This makes massaging too tiring. The masseur also needs to be comfortable and supported, so that all their energies can go into the massage, and not into supporting themselves.

If the patient is sitting on a chair, the masseur also sits on a chair, so that they are at the right height for massaging.

If the patient needs a bed, choose the bed , (hoping that you have a choice), which is at the right height for the masseur. A higher bed is better. A very low divan necessitates a stoop from the masseur, and they won't be able to stoop for long without their own back hurting! If the bed is not suitable, try the floor. With the patient on the floor, again supported with pillows, the masseur kneels down beside them. A cushion for the masseur's knees makes it more comfortable.

MASSAGE

What are the actual massage movements?

The following massage movements can be done by the patient themselves or their masseur. Which ever technique is used, remember that the aim is to induce relaxation in the muscle.

How deep do you do the massage?

This depends on the patient.

Some prefer very, very gentle massage. Some prefer the massage to be quite deep.

Who decides which is right? —— the patients, it is their pain and they have to do the relaxation. So whichever technique they choose, it is the right one for them at that time. They should feel the massage, but it should never be painful.

There are several massage techniques. Here are a few easy ones to learn:

a) *Stroking*. Place the whole hand on the patient and stroke the skin fairly firmly, rather like stroking the cat. If it is a big area, like the back, both hands can work together. If it is a small area, like the arm or neck, the hands can work one at a time. The hands can move forwards, or backwards, or from side to side. This can continue, but vary the movements.

b) *Finger massage*. Place the pads of all four fingers on the area. Keep the fingers together. Press, and make small circles. Keep your fingers in touch with the patient's skin, so that their skin moves with your fingers. Don't simply rub the skin. Don't dig your finger nails in. Make six circles. Move your fingers to another area and make another six circles and so on.

c) *Finger spread massage.* Place the hand flat on the area. Press slightly. Spread the fingers and thumb out, keeping in touch with the skin. Bring fingers and thumb together, keeping the fingers straight. When bringing the fingers and thumb together, the natural action is to raise the knuckles and palm. This is the correct movement. Repeat this six times. Move your hand to a nearby area and repeat.

d) *Finger pressure.* Place the fingers on a tender spot. Press. Hold it there for five seconds. Meanwhile the patient breathes with his diaphragm. Release the pressure.

Some patients find that this numbs the pain and they like it. Some patients do not like it, so don't do it for them.

e) *Knuckle massage.* Make a fist of your hand. Place the knuckles on the area. Press gently in. Make six circular movements. Then move your knuckles to a nearby area and make another six circular movements and so on. This is quite a useful technique if your fingers start to ache during the massage.

This massage is performed as deeply as the patient wants.

How do we know how deep to do the massage?

I suggest that you only press very lightly to begin with. Then increase the pressure bit by bit. Ask the patient which is the most comfortable depth.

Some patients can hardly bare you to touch them, because the pain is so severe. So only do very light stroking to them.

Some patients benefit from deep massage. So do any of the above strokes with some pressure. But don't be rough. Be firm and slow.

Some patients may even like to use the edge of a door for massage! If the pain is in the middle of the back between the shoulder blades, and therefore difficult to massage themselves, they open a door. They stand with their back to the door, hold the handles to steady it, and rub the door on their back muscles. Rather like a bull rubbing his neck on the fence post. Some patients really like this! and it can be effective.

Finally, remember, the aim of massage is to help promote relaxation of the muscles.

It can be done by the patient themselves.

It can be done by a relative or friend.

Whether it is light gentle massage, or deep massage, this is determined by the patients themselves.

Chapter 24
Questions

1) Why is backache so painful after sitting?

Because when we are sitting there is nothing to stop the muscles tensing. On the other hand when we are moving about, the muscles are made to contract and to a small extent, relax. There is also, an improved blood supply available when we move.

2) Why are tense muscles so painful first thing in the morning after a night's rest?

There are two reasons for this:

a) After the tension of the previous day, there is an excess of lactic acid in the muscles which keeps the muscles shortened, (see chapter 10), even if you are good at relaxing and have had a good night's rest.

b) Waking up is a gradual process. In sleep the heart beats slower, respiration is slower and more shallow. As we waken, our heart and breathing quicken back to normal, the brain starts thinking and 'worrying' and the associated muscle tension occurs. By the time we open our eyes, our muscles are tense to the point of pain.

3) If the pain wakes me in the middle of the night, what do I do?

If it wakes you in the middle of the night, the pain is obviously severe. It's no good saying 'relax and go to sleep', because it does not work. You need to get up. You won't want to, but if you lie in bed you won't sleep anyway. So you might as well get up, move around, refill the hot water bottle, then go back to bed and place it by the sore part and relax.

4) Can sleeping awkwardly give me neck pain?

Unlikely. Take the example of falling asleep in a train. Your head lolls over and when you wake up you have got a stiff neck, but after a bit of movement, all stiffness goes. The pain does not last all day. If you sleep awkwardly in bed, you may have a temporary pain but it disappears after a bit of movement.

5) Do I have to put a board under the mattress?

No. An ordinary firm mattress is all that is necessary.

If the mattress sags right down then a board may be of some use, but it only solves half the problem and you should really get a new mattress and bed.

6) Does sitting in a draught make my painful neck worse?

Yes. Cold makes all matter contract, including muscles. So in cold and damp weather, the tense muscles increase their tension and so the pain is worse. Heat makes all matter expand and so helps to elongate the muscle, and thus ease the pain. Heat, such as a hot bath, hot water bottle, or heat lamp, directed on to the painful muscles increases the blood supply, which helps to neutralise excessive lactic acid, (see chapter 10), so again helping the muscle to attain its natural length and ease the pain.

7) Is my headache caused by tense muscles?

It can be.

If your Occipito Frontalis muscle, which lies under your scalp, is tense, you will have a headache.

8) Why is sneezing so painful?

A sneeze causes a convulsive action of the body, forcing the muscles to contract hard. Unfortunately, this sometimes makes the muscles in your neck and particularly your back, increase their tension and therefore the pain.

9) I am overweight. Does it matter?

All people including those who are overweight, can suffer muscle pain from stress.

It makes no difference. However, if you are overweight, you may need to lose some weight for your general health.

10) Why can I play sport without pain and yet, while I'm relaxing watching television, it can be extremely painful?

There are two reasons for this:

a) You probably enjoy your sport and are able to 'switch off' from the stresses of life. The television, on the other hand, is not totally absorbing. You watch the television, but maybe you are bored with it, and so you think of everything else, including any stress in your life. With the stress, the muscle tenses and so the pain occurs.

b) The movement of the body in sport brings more blood to the muscles which helps to neutralise the excess lactic acid, (see chapter 10). This is not happening when you are sitting watching the television.

11) Is it psycho-somatic?

No. Psycho-somatic, these days, is used to describe the symptoms of patients, who are considered to be imagining them in order to gain sympathy or attention. *This has absolutely nothing to do with the condition described in this book.* As a matter of fact, imagining a pain by itself will not induce muscle tension leading to genuine pain.

12) Can I prevent it from coming on?

No. As the muscle tension caused by Body Language is a natural and subconscious reaction it will occur, even though we understand the reasons. Having said that, if it does 'just come on', you should now know the correct course of action to take from the very beginning. From experience, patients who know the correct course of action to take still get neck or backache, or pain in other parts of the body, but now they can handle it by following the explanation, guidance and instructions in this book. After all, the author sometimes suffers!

Chapter 25
Summary

1) As a reaction to stress, or to a 'problem' in life, the muscles in the body tense. Sometimes this is visible to the eye and is called Body Language. Sometimes only part of a muscle tenses and it is not visible.

2) This is a normal reaction, it is a reflex and is totally subconscious.

3) The muscles that tense depend on the person's reaction to the stress. Different reactions bring about different Body Language. Different Body Language uses different muscles.

4) Tense muscles which *remain tense, become painful*.

5) Treatment is aimed at relaxing the muscles and, when required, addressing the stress.

6) However, a complete cure will *only* be effected if:

   a) the source of stress is removed, or

   b) the person changes their attitude towards the stress, so that it is no longer a stress to them, or

   c) they forget it completely.

How to use this book
(for people who read books backwards)

The book covers most parts of the body.

To get the full understanding of the sequence by which pain is the result of muscle tension, caused by Body Language, which itself is the result of stress, first read chapters 1 to 12. This will greatly help you in dealing with your specific problem. It is true that chapters 1 to 12 talk about pain in the neck and back only. Don't let this put you off. The mechanism as to how the pain is produced applies to backs and necks and to other parts of the body. So read these chapters first, and then the chapter that particularly interests you.

For example: if tennis elbow is the problem, read chapters 1 to 12, then read the chapter on tennis elbow. So for:

Necks and Backs	Chapters 1 to 16
Tennis Elbow	Chapters 1 to 12 then Chapters 17 and 18
Shoulder	Chapters 1 to 12 then Chapters 17 and 19
Chest wall	Chapters 1 to 12 then Chapters 17 and 20
Front of the ribs	Chapters 1 to 12 then Chapters 17 and 21
Front of the thighs and groin	Chapters 1 to 12 then Chapters 17 and 22

Then, finally, read the Summary in Chapter 25.

Bibliography

Bogduk, N. and Twomey, L.T. (1991). *Clinical Anatomy of the Lumbar Spine*, 2nd ed., Churchill Livingstone, Singapore.

Daniels, L., Williams, M., Worthingham, C. (1947). *Muscle Testing*. W.B.Saunders Company.

Draspa, L.J. (1959). 'Psychological Factors in Muscular Pain'. *British Journal of Medical Psychology,* 32, 106.

Draspa, L.J. (1961). 'A Behavioural Investigation into Muscular Pain'. *Psychiatria et Neurologia*, Basel, 141, 367.

Draspa, L.J. (1961). 'Neuro-physiological Mechanisms involved in Muscular Pain'. *Psychiatria et Neurologia,* Basel, 141, 202.

Draspa, J. (1970). 'The Treatment of Muscular Pain resulting from Covert Behaviour.' *Physiotherapy*, 56, 548.

Draspa, J. (1986). 'Stress and Pain'. *In Touch. The Journal of the Organisation of Chartered Physiotherapists in Private Practice*, 42, 16.

Gray's Anatomy, (1980). Longmans.

McKenzie, Robin. (1985). *Treat Your Own Back*, Spinal Publications Ltd.